VITAMINS & MINERALS
FROM A TO Z

Compiled & Written by
JEWEL POOKRUM, M.D., Ph.D.

A&B BOOKS PUBLISHERS
Brooklyn, New York
11201

Vitamins and Minerals From A to Z. ©1993 By Jewel Pookrum. Printed and bound in the United States of America. All rights reserved. No part of this book may be reproduced in any form or by any means including electronic, mechanical or photocopying or stored in a retrieval system without permission in writing from the publisher except by a reviewer who may quote brief passage to be included in a review.

Published by *A&B BOOKS PUBLISHERS* 149 Lawrence St. Brooklyn, NY 11201 (718) 596-3389 by arrangements with J.E.W.E.L Publications 60 East Ferry St., Detroit, Michigan.

The contents of this book are for the purposes of education and information and is not intended to be a substitute for medical supervision

Library of Congress Cataloging- in -Publication Data

Pookrum, Jewel.
   Vitamins and Minerals from A to Z / compiled written by Jewel Pookrum.
      p.   cm.
  ISBN: 1-881316-66-1
    formerly
  ISBN: 1-83104-00-9
  Includes bibliographical references and index.
  1.Vitamins in human nutrition.   2. Minerals in human nutrition.
I. Title.
RA784. P65   1993   93-46568
612. 3' 99 --dc20.   CIP

COVER DESIGN: *A & B BOOKS PUBLISHERS*
ILLUSTRATION: *MSHINDO I.*

96 95 94 93   4 3 2 1
Printed in the United States

DEDICATION

This humble work is dedicated to the Source from which it comes,

YAHWEH,

the Creator of all things

I lovingly thank my mother, children and friends for being a nourishing source of inspiration, which has prompted me to share YAHWEH's truth in writing.

Always and with love!

Dr. Jewel Pookrum, M.D. Ph. D
J.E.W.E.L. PUBLICATIONS

SYNOPSIS

Many people are perplexed about vitamins:
1) What are they for?
2) How are they to be used? and
3) From what sources should they come?

This manual gives the reader a complete guideline course on how to use vitamins along with a clear description of their function. This manual will also instruct you as to how each vitamin and mineral discussed can be identified in foods. Discussed also in some detail is the ethnicity of race, especially the melanin-dominant race and how minerals and vitamins are applicable to this majority population on planet Earth.

TABLE OF CONTENTS

DEDICATION..
SYNOPSIS..
INTRODUCTION.. 1
ETHNICITY.. 7
MELANIN.. 19
LIGHT AND HEALTH 33
VITAMINS.. 61
   VITAMIN A (BETA CAROTENE)...................... 61
   VITAMIN C (Ascorbic ACID) 64
   VITAMIN D 69
   VITAMIN E... 72
   VITAMIN K 74
   VITAMIN B.. 76
      Vitamin B-Complex 76
      Vitamin B1 (Thiamine) 76
      Vitamin B2 (RIBOFLAVIN) 77
      Vitamin B3 (NIACIN, Niacinamide) 81
      Pantothenic ACID (B5) 83
      Vitamin B6 (Pyridoxine) 84
      VITAMIN B12 (Cyanocobalamin) 86
   BIOTIN... 88
   CHOLINE 91
   FOLIC ACID.. 93
   INOSITOL 95
   PARA-AMINOBENZOIC ACID (PABA).................. 96
   BIOFLAVONOIDS.. 97
NUTRIENTS & DOSAGES FOR MAINTAINING GOOD HEALTH 101
MINERALS... 107
   Calcium... 109
   Iron 113
   Zinc 115
   Copper 116

Selenium	118
Aluminum	118
Gold	121
HALOGENS	**125**
Fluorine	125
Iodine	126
SUMMARY	**129**
REFERENCES	**130**
GLOSSARY	**131**
INDEX	**138**

INTRODUCTION

Dr. Jewel: Having been trained to be a surgeon, a medical doctor, hematologist and a practitioner of psychoneuro immunologic medicine, have given me an opportunity to be able to observe many aspects of what being a human is all about.

I have had many personal experiences that have allowed me to be really thankful and recognize that my existence as a human being on this planet at this very moment is truly a divine gift and a treasure of information that is available to all of us from all dimensions. Truly, each and everyone of us is a god and goddess, gifted with a divine gift and talent and a true sincere and infinite love that will regenerate and renew any area, any aspect of our life within our physical, mental, and spiritual existence.

"Vitamins and Minerals from A to Z" is truly a gift that has come through me to remind myself and all of my African Ancestry of the divine gift that has been given to us in the form of Being exactly who we are, Africans. Many days I spent eight to ten hours of my life wading in the abdominal and pelvic regions of many people's bodies. No person is exactly the same inside. Yes, we all have livers, we all have lungs, we all have hearts, we all have arteries and the like. However, the branching, the size, shape, color, the degree of function and too often the location, varies extremely from individual to individual, sex to sex and definitely from race to race.

Dr. Roger Williams was one of the scientific intellectuals who wrote an entire book entitled

"Biochemical Individuality". Within this treatise he identified that chemically each individual is different. Each family differs from another family.

In my disillusionment of seeing my own people suffer in the large institutions we have in America known as hospitals, it became a nightmare to try to understand why, with the vast degree of technology that we have, that the African male life span is short, that the morbidity and the mortality rate for an African newborn is so high, that the rate of hysterectomy and sterilization is continuously rising in the African woman as compared to other races. Was it really true that we had weaker genes? Was it really true that our varied economic state played a significant role in the decline of our health ? The answer is no.

What I discovered in my search to identify myself and why we failed to respond to a medical system in which I was taught had all the answers, was the simple fact that the standard of evaluating the health of the patient was never a standard based on the patient's anatomy, physiology, growth and development curves. When I came into the awareness that the western medical standard of health chemically is based on the blood chemistry of the Caucasian male and female, and the physiology and anatomy of the Caucasian male and female, it was quite obvious that I could never experience optimal health care when measured by a standard that belongs to another race.

I became real enraged and I wondered how could this be, how could I be standing in the middle of a hospital that has 1300 beds, 99 percent of them occupied by Africans and the standard to measure whether the blood count was normal, whether the urinalysis was normal is based on a Caucasian Chemistry. To maintain a sense of well being and peace in my body, I immediately look desperately for the answers. The first thing I looked to was economics which brought truly a peace and a realization of the need to understand the historic "God Bless the child that has his own" concept.

When I recognize that all the hospitals in America have been created by profit or non-profit monies from Caucasians with the intent that they or their family members will be able to receive ideal health care, would it not stand to reason that if one built the hospital, if one was responsible for supplying all of the instruments and the bedding for the hospital, that the standard to determine whether one was healthy or not would be a standard that was based on the founders' innate chemistry and make up. Had Africans collectively put their monies together to build a hospital, to build research laboratories, to build medical investigatory companies to identify our standard blood chemistry, our standard growth curves, the true values needed that would benefit our race family - may be institutionalized. So, the only thing that I could really gripe about was the fact that the hospitals in America and in the western world in general market themselves as being able to render health care to all races. However, they never ask you to read the implied small print, which infers: that the Caucasians are the ones that finance the hospital so they will always be the standard. Is that mis-marketing or is that a lack of astuteness on our part not to investigate what is the standard that is being used to determine whether I as an African woman am healthy or not?

Is that not the question I should ask when I go into the hospital because that is the question I should ask when I go to the shoe store, do you have my size? That is the question that I ask when I go grocery shopping do you have what I want? I have not been able to elucidate why the African does not ask this same question when we are purchasing health care. Is my laboratory test determination based on a population of individuals who are like myself ?. For whatever reason, we do not ask the question and therefore we do get the answer. Therefore, we do not get the best treatment.

Vitamins and Minerals from A to Z is the first of many series that I am writing to inform myself: which is all of my people about our uniqueness as a race within the family of humans. To bring to our awareness, the developmental curves, the nutritional needs and our inherited cultural values which are responsible for making us the unique Being that we are!.

If we are to be the best that we have been created to be, then we must be willing to do the research and the investigation. Most of all we must be willing to invest the money and create the time necessary to know who we were historically and where we are in the present, so we can determine how we want to enter the future.

I hope you will enjoy this information and if you learn nothing else from reading this book I wish that you too clearly understand from this day on that the well known "One a day Vitamins" is not a vitamin that can accurately supplement the proper diet for a melanin dominant male, female or child.

Ethnicity

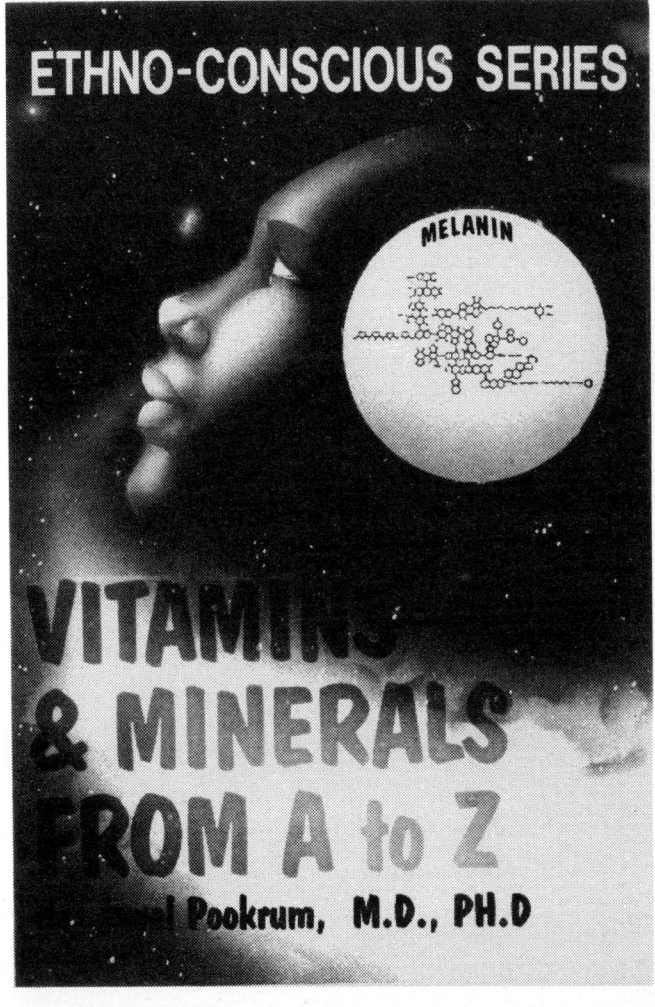

ETHNICITY

It is important to remember that every living organism requires the "Life Force Energy" to sustain itself. The questions of how much, when, and under what circumstances are very important to answer in order to maintain the distinct character and function (purpose) of each species. Among humans, each race has specific distinctions and functions that are paramount for a healthy and balanced relationship with other humans and planet Earth. Each race must honor and respect its own uniqueness to remain healthy and functional within its race.

At the present time, the needs and distinctions of the Caucasian race have dominated the world and set the standards for health. This has created much misinformation in the races as to what is best for them health-wise to maintain balance. The misapplication of Caucasian health needs to non-Caucasian races has resulted in the near extinction of the native American Indian, the Eskimo, the Australian Aborigine and many other species of the non-Caucasian human race.

Researchers like Dr. Stanley Garn, a professor of Human Nutrition at the School of Public Health and a Professor of Anthropology, The University of Michigan, Ann Arbor, Michigan, U.S.A., have been very concerned since the mid-1960s of the possible sequel " the mis-determination of one race status by another race's standards.[1] "

The magnitude and implication of apparent race differences in hemoglobin values, published in the American Journal of Clinical Nutrition, 1975[2] makes it clear that the differences in blood composition and content in various races is a genetic standard and to assume the variation is pathological when compared to another race's blood values and would ensue action nutritional and otherwise that may be lethal to the racial group assumed to be pathologic.

Research upon and the collection of data from large racial populations, consistently verifies that each race family has its own growth rate variation, blood values, bone and neurologic development curves, confirming the uniqueness of each race.

Since the major and largest population of humans on the planet is melanin-dominant (black/brown-skinned), we will describe the main features or uniqueness of the dominant race on planet Earth before proceeding with our treatise on minerals and vitamins and their food sources.

Developmental Differences

Females of any race are developmentally more advanced over boys, even at birth. Thus the neonatal survival rate is greater for any female of any race. Extensive research reveals that the melanin dominant

---

[1] Vergheses, K.P., et al: Studies in Growth and Development XII. "Physical Growth of North American Negro children", Pediatrics 44:243-247, 1969.

[2] Wingerd, J. Schoen, E,S. Solomon, I. L ,: Growth Standards in the First Two Years of Life based on Measurements of White and Black Children in a Prepaid Health Care Program. Pediatrics 47:818-825, 1971.

infant is developmentally Advanced neurologically and integumentally (skin and hair).[3] Melanin dominant neonates weight less and are shorter at birth as compared to melanin recessive neonates. "These dimensional differences are reversed within the next three years of life. From the second year of life through age 14, melanin dominant boys and girls stand taller and hormonal sexual development is advanced over their melanin recessive age peers."[4]

Dental Advancement

Melanin-dominant children exhibit earlier dental development (permanent tooth eruption) than their melanin recessive counterparts. The eruption of 28 out of 32 permanent teeth occurs earlier in the melanin dominant child. Bone and Tooth development are advanced in melanin dominant children irregardless of the socio-economic status of the family. American Black children evidently grow faster and are skeletally and dentally advanced during the first decade and beyond."[5]

Infants

Black infants are smaller in weight and length at birth than Caucasian infants, and at the same time developmentally advanced when the infants are born full-term and mothers have received standard

---

[3] Owen, G.M & A.H. Lubin: Anthropometric differences between Black and White preschool children. Am.J. Diseases of Children, 126: 168-169, 1973.

[4] Wingerd, J., I. L. Solomon & E.J. Schoen: Parent-Specific height standards for Preadolescent children of the three racial groups with method of rapid determination. Pediatrics 52:556-560, 1973.

[5] Garn, S.M., Tendency towards greater stature in American Black children. Am. J. Diseases of children, 126: 164-166, 1973.

prenatal care. During the childhood and adolescent years, the melanin-dominant girl and boy stand taller than Caucasian girls and boys of the same age group. This indicates that nutritional requirements must be balanced and present during the childhood and teen years of the melanin-dominant children to provide for the accelerated growth spurt experienced during this phase of development. Studies also show that the adult stature of the melanin-dominant male and female is attained at an earlier age (in mid-teens) than is that of Caucasian teenagers.

Conclusion

Some portion of Black children who are actually at a nutritional risk may appear both satisfactory, and even normal, if White developmental nutritional standards are employed.

HEMATOLOGICAL DIFFERENCES

The measurement of the hemoglobin concentration (mg/100 ML) and of the hematocrit (packed red-cell volume) has long been a useful part of nutritional assessment. We have evidence that "normal values" are not the same for melanin-dominant races and Caucasians. This statement is based on a study of more than 100,000 determinations. Overall, the differences are of the order of 1.0 gm/100 ml for hemoglobin concentrations, and three percent (3%) in the hematocrit (packed red-cell volume). It exists at all ages, from infancy through the 7th decade of life and in melanin-dominant males and females alike. It exists even at high levels of reported Iron intake, in athletes whose tests indicate higher hemoglobin and hematocrit values, in pregnant women (in the first and second trimesters), and in infants supplemented for the first 18 months.

Research has also noted that among adult melanin-dominant males and females, the White blood cell count is lower by almost 500 to 1,000 cells and the T-4 cell count is also lower.

SUMMARY

The implications of nutritional surveys and nutritional assessments seem clear. Equally low hemoglobins do not have the same nutritional implications in both melanin-dominant and Caucasian individuals; the cut-off value should not be the same. In view of what we now know about hemoglobin and hematocrit alike, there is reason for population- standards.

It is noted that if melanin-dominant boys and girls are both taller than Caucasian boys and girls and developmentally advanced, their 1.00 gm/100 ml poor hemoglobin is not indicative of poorer nutritional status. It is their norm.

DIFFERENCES AND SKELETAL MASS

From the fetal period onward through childhood and into old age, individuals of the melanin-dominant race and ancestries have 1) a greater skeletal mass, 2) a larger mineral mass, and 3) a higher whole bone density. This statement is based upon studies of fetal skeletons, skeletalized material of both sexes, and finally, on X-ray evaluations of over 26,000 melanin-dominant people.

This population difference in the magnitude of the skeletal mass and the mineral mass has major implications in the nutritional diagnosis, especially for the diagnosis of metabolic disorders involving the skeletal mass and the interpretation of adult "osteoporosis," and in the osteodystrophies of kidney origin.

One of the clinical manifestations of protein-calorie malnutrition, by way of example, is a diminution in the mineral mass both in childhood protein-calorie malnutrition and adult protein-calorie malnutrition, to nothing of adult malabsorption states. With a greater skeletal mass at all ages, the use of Caucasian norms for a melanin-dominant skeletal and mineral mass would conceal bone losses long after the bone losses were clinically present.

A similar problem of ours is that in other bone-losing situations, including the osteodystrophies of renal origin, using techniques other than X-rays, when chronic renal disease patients are studied whether they be transplant patients or dialyzed patients two general observations may always be made. First, the chronic renal disease patient evidenced considerable bone loss. Second, despite the bone loss that has obviously occurred, age, sex, and treatment matched melanin-dominant patients show systematically more bone than the patients who are Caucasian. The larger skeletal mass of American melanin-dominant people compared with the Caucasian norms showed the need for norms that are not just equal but bigger in regard to calcium and protein requirements.

SOURCES FOR PROTEIN AND MINERALS FOR MELANIN-DOMINANT INDIVIDUALS

Previous reading has indicated there are obvious nutritional needs for the melanin-dominant race that are distinct from the Caucasian race. However, it is very important to note that the food substances selected to supply these additional needs have to be scrutinized very closely. The Caucasian race uses animal flesh as a major source of protein and minerals. By appearances, this has been an adequate source of these nutrients for this population. However, aging diseases and many other physical deformities still occur with the selection of flesh as a major source for meeting nutritional requirements. Man originated from the melanin-dominant race, and examined skeletal structures indicate that the teeth of this early man were suited to eating plants. This supports the idea that the genetic information in the melanin-dominant body is programmed for vegetable consumption as a source of protein and minerals, not flesh. As more melanin-dominant people begin to digest flesh as a source of protein, mineral blockage diseases become major problems. Typical blockage diseases include hypertension, diabetes, arthritis, gout, obesity, coronary heart disease and eye diseases. Blockage diseases eventually lead to deficiency diseases because normal pathways to take in nutrients are blocked; therefore, deficiencies eventually ensue.

Summary

The evidence accumulated so far underscores identifiable differences between melanin-dominant Americans and Caucasian Americans that are crucial in the nutritional assessments and to the measurement of nutritional status. Given such differences in the skeletal mass, hemoglobin and hematocrit concentrations, it is not appropriate to measure one group's status by another group's standards. These are not differences brought about by poverty or the lack of privilege, but rather, they are fundamental differences (related to ethnic origin) that we cannot afford to neglect. Note: it is very important for the melanin-dominant individual to study this material so that he/she can ensure that one's treating physician, nurse, or nutritionist is aware of this information so as to make recommendations for dietary guidelines, pharmaceutical guidelines, exercise guidelines, etc., that are based on your distinct needs. If your physician, nutritionist or nurse says that there is no such thing or uses the term "we are all the same," or that these differences are not important, then get a second, third, or fourth opinion until one finds a professional who is able to treat the melanin-dominant individual as his/her body needs specify. Any gardener knows that he cannot raise violets like chrysanthemums. Each race has to honor its own distinct nutritional requirements and medical needs. While we are all of one race (the human race), there are distinctions that allow us to remain unique and contributory.

REFERENCES

Garn, Stanley M., Ph.D. and D.C. Clark, *Problems in the Nutritional Assessment of Black Individuals* AJPH March, 1976, Vol. 66, No. 3.

Gonz, S.M., G.M. Owens and D.C. Clark, AMERICAN JOURNAL OF PHARMACOLOGY, Vol. 66, No. 3, March 1976.

THE QUESTION OF RACE DIFFERENCE IN STATUTE NORMS. E: ECOL. Food Nutr, Food: 319-327.

Wingerd, J., I.L. Solomon, and E.J. Schaea. SPECIFIC HEALTH STANDARDS FOR PRE-ADOLESCENT CHILDREN OF THREE RACES. Pediatrics 52: 556-560, 1973.

Stewart, N.A., Ph.D., MELANIN AND SENSORY-MOTOR DEVELOPMENT IN THE AFRICAN INFANT; ASSESSMENT IMPLICATIONS. (1980). Thesis.

Reed, T.E. CAUCASIAN GENES IN AMERICAN
    NEGROES. Science 165, 762=768, 1969.

Hiernaux, J. ETHNIC DIFFERENCES IN GROWTH AND
    DEVELOPMENT. Eugen. Quart. 15, 12-21,
    1968.

Tanner, J.M. GROWTH AND ADOLESCENCE, 2nd ed.
    Blackwell, Oxford, 1962.

Garn, S.M. HUMAN RACE, 3rd ed. Thomas,
    Springfield, IL., 1971.

Garn, S.M. PHYSICAL GROWTH AND
DEVELOPMENT. Am. J. Phys. Anthrop. 10, 169-192,
1952.

Garn, S.M., N.J. Smith and D.C. Clark. Race
    differences in hemoglobin levels. Ecol. Food
Nutr. 3: 299-301, 1974

Garn, S.M. N.J. smith and D.C. Clark.
    Long differences in hemoglobin leaves between
    blacks and whites. J. Natl. Med. Assoc. 67:91-96,
    1975
    Owens. G.M., and A.H Lubin. Anthropometeric
    differences between black and whites preschool
    children Am. J. Dis. Child. 126:168-169, 1973

Melanin

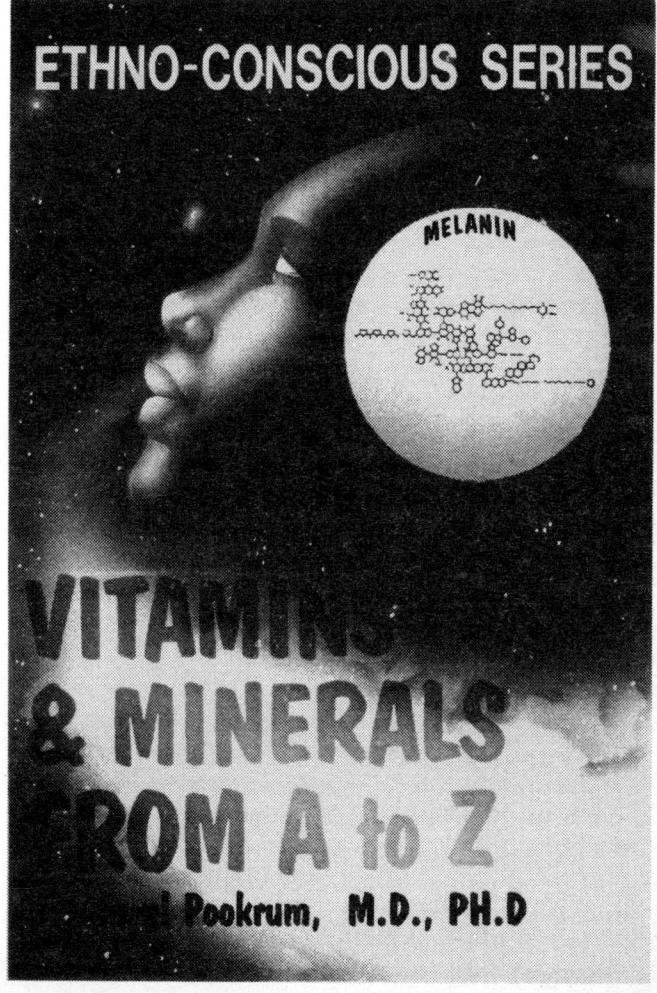

MELANIN

Upon studying the previous chapter, it is obvious that the genetic structure of individuals definitely will determine their physiological need for certain food substances and will also determine the types of vitamins and minerals necessary to allow individuals to maintain their own unique function. As we continue to investigate the diversity and genetic distinction among race, the need for specific nutrients based on their unique genetic structure becomes apparent. When evaluating the nutritional needs of the melanin-dominant race, it is obvious that the pigmentation of these identified individuals is not just surface pigmentation throughout the skin, hair and irises of the eyes, but also is found within the very cell structures of the internal organs. This pigment we have identified as giving the appearance of color is the variation of a substance known as melanin.

The word "melanin" comes from the Greek word for black. Melanin is a pigment that ranges in color from pale yellow through reddish brown to blue black. It is also in almost every major organ of the body. One of its major purposes is to shield and protect body tissue against radiation damage.

Melanin in its most concentrated and purest form is black. It is black because its chemical structure will not allow any type of energy to escape once that energy has come into contact with it. There are multiple chemical reactions that happen within the melanin molecule that allow it to have total energy-saving efficiency. When these reactions are completed within the melanin molecule, no energy is reflected away from the surface of the molecule structure. In order for this molecule to be an energy-efficient and energy-saving entity, the molecule requires reactions with substances such as amino acids, minerals, and particular vitamins for that efficiency.

It is obvious that individuals who have little or no melanin would not require the same amount of the specific minerals and vitamins as individuals who are intensely melanin-dominant (MD). This obviously indicates that the nutritional needs of these two individuals, just based upon their melanin content, would be significantly different. Minerals and vitamins that would maintain a melanin-recessive metabolism in its normal state would not be adequate for the melanin-dominant individual. MD individuals, possessing greater quantities of melanin within their bodies, would require specific, different, and more of certain nutrients to maintain normal melanin function.

We will look more in depth at melanin later and describe additional nutrients necessary for melanin's optimal activity. Before we describe these components, however, let us get a better understanding of just what melanin does.

It is important to understand that matter, because of its molecular composition, does not reflect light from its surface, that the object regardless of what it is, will appear black in color. When an object does reflect energy or light from its surface, the light that is reflected determines its color.

For example, if all the energy is reflected from the surface of an object, that object will appear white. If an object appears to be red, it is absorbing all energy around it except the red energy, which is being reflected away from the object. The eye captures (absorbs) the red light that is reflected and processes it so that the brain perceives that particular energy as the color red.

Melanin and melanin health have a direct relationship with light exposure and light captivity. Light energy from natural sources such as the sun or certain artificial sources cause melanin to be black in color.

Let us look a little more into the physics of light. When a light wave leaves the sun or your stereo, because you must remember that sound waves are a form of light, it travels in space until it comes in contact with a melanin structure in the skin. Melanin, through its internal reaction system, then stores this energy and reflects very little of it away from itself, causing a visual reaction of blackness.

Melanin may be viewed as a battery that is partially charged and can always accept any electrical charge. When energy is captured, the melanin battery has more energy to utilize in metabolism and memory processes. Melanin obtains this energy free charge directly from its surroundings. This means that melanin-dominant individuals can charge up their melanin just by being in the sun or around the right type of musical sounds or other energy sources.

On the microscopic level, the melanin molecules rearrange themselves and undergo what is known as "resonance". Resonance is the capacity to move back and forth at a certain rate in space and time. This resonance or rearrangement of the electrons causes the structures of these electrons to be able to hold much more energy as they vibrate back and forth within the melanin molecule. Visualize little Styrofoam balls being charged with energy. They jump up and down like popcorn. As they continue to do that, they will begin to move faster and faster with the increased heat they absorb.

It is important to know that melanin is charged and activated by the following forms of electromagnetic energy:

Sound, radio, TV waves, microwaves, thermal radiant heat, visible light, x-rays, cosmic rays, ultraviolet light and the earth's magnetic energy. All charge melanin and cause it to absorb energy and store that energy and pass the stored energy on to other cells in the body so that they can charge and regenerate themselves.

THE PRODUCTION OF MELANIN BY THE BODY

Melanin is synthesized and distributed by specialized cells, known as melanocytes, within the organs of the body. Melanocytes synthesize melanin through a series of biochemical reactions beginning with the intake of the amino acid phenylalanine. Each step in the production of melanin requires certain nutritional components and particular minerals and vitamins, including B vitamins, pyrodoxine, copper, riboflavin, pantothenic acid, tyrosine and/or phenylalanine. Each biochemical reaction in the chain is controlled by a specific enzyme. If all the essential enzymes, vitamins and minerals are present, the pigment melanin is produced in considerable quantities. Melanin is produced and the individual has dark skin, black hair, and brown eyes. If any of the enzymes or nutrients are deficient or relatively inactive, the individual manifests a pale skin color. Hair will be light or blond, and eyes will be hazel or blue. The occurrence of a state of depigmentation is directly related to the genetic inability to produce sufficient amounts of melanin.

Melanin is produced not only by melanocytes; melanin has been discovered in and found to be produced by mast cells, which are a component of the blood stream. At present, the reason for melanin production in the mast cells is not clear. Melanin is also produced in the nervous system and brain, but without the aid of melanocytes.

TYPES OF MELANIN

Melanin is always contained in a small battery cell known as a melanosome. Melanosomes are contained within the larger cell structure of melanin known as a melanocyte. The degree of blackness of various organs or melanin centers throughout the body of the melanin-dominant individual depends upon catalyst concentration, catalyst chemical reactivity or catalyst electrical charge, and the type of melanin and its weight.

There are three major types of melanin. Eumelanin, which has a very high electrical charge, is quite concentrated in its molecular weight and density, and is extremely absorbent. It gives the appearance of the colors of dark brown to blue black. A less dense form of melanin with a lower molecular weight and less capacity to absorb and store energy is known as pheo-melanin or pseudo-melanin. Pheo-melanin gives more of the yellowish brown and slightly reddish tints to the skin and hair. It has been determined that individuals with no melanin have far more cancers and genetic disorders than do individuals possessing pheo-melanin. It has also been identified that individuals possessing pheo-melanin have more diseases, disorders and genetic deformities than do individuals possessing eumelanin.

Six types of melanin have been identified and classified from one to six based on concentration and activity. Type 1 individuals usually have white skin and produce very little melanin. They have blue eyes, blond or very red hair and often have freckles. They have a Celtic background and usually originate from Irish, Scottish, or Welsh groups.

Melanin Types 2 and 3 are also associated with what anthropologists identify as the Caucasian race. Type 4 individuals, however, are lightly tanned, and their skin color ranges from pale yellow to a ruddy red. Japanese, Chinese, Italians, Greeks, Spanish and Red Indians belong to this type. Their production of pheo-melanin is of a moderate level, and they present a moderate risk for the development of skin disorders and organ imbalances.

Types 5 and 6 individuals range from brown skinned to very black-skinned. Type 5 melanin is found in ethnic groups such as Mexicans, Malaysians, Puerto Ricans, and certain other Spanish speaking people.

Type 6, or true eumelanin, is found in Egyptians, Ethiopians, Nigerians, American Africans and Australian aborigines. They always have black hair and very dark brown to black eyes. Their incidence of skin abnormalities and other aging phenomena is very rare and slow to develop under normal conditions.

One of the main nutrients that is a precursor or foundation for melanin production is tyrosine. The body must contain the enzyme known as tyrosine and copper to be able to utilize tyrosine to produce melanin. We can see that the melanin-dominant individual has a definite need for certain amino acids (when compared to other individuals) and definitely requires certain mineral nutrients at a higher concentration than those who are melanin-recessive.

There are four primary pathways that can produce melanin with the use of different amino acids and breakdown products from amino Acid activity. Foods that have been identified as containing the amino acids phenylalanine; or tyrosine will always provide the initial building blocks for melanin. These foods include bananas, grapes, mushrooms, and dark green leafy vegetables.

PROPERTIES OF MELANIN

Melanin has a number of interesting properties that are already known to the scientific community. Please study very closely the following attributes of melanin:

1. Melanin can become toxic to MD people if it combines with harmful drugs, amphetamines, psychotic hallucinogens such as LSD, neuroleptics known as tranquilizers, marijuana, Agent Orange, paraquats (usually associated with marijuana), and tetracycline.

2. Melanin shows extreme affinity for binding with fatty type compounds; therefore, the more MD individuals are, the greater affinity they have to retain excess fat in the body or store fats taken in from the diet. Wesson oil, sunflower seed oil, corn oil these oils have a structure within them that makes them compatible to binding with melanin. This can be a dangerous factor when we eat fats that have saturated bonds within them. The saturated fatty acids (as we call them) can create hardening of the arteries at a much greater rate in individuals who are MD. Therefore, the ingestion of animal fat can create hardening of the arteries when consumed by MD individuals.

3. Melanin is a very old chemical and has been involved in the life process since life began. It is composed of varying amounts of different small chemical species and nutritional substances known as tyrosine, tryptophan, melatonin, and serotonin. You will note that two of these substances are essential amino acids.

4. Melanin exhibits varying types of electrical charges and binding properties responsible for its great electromagnetic and electric activity.

5. Melanin responds to and absorbs light, sound (in the form of music) and electrical energy, and uses this energy in the body as food, as a nutrient. It converts light energy to sound energy and back again to light energy. Melanin is an extremely stable chemical and is very difficult to analyze in laboratory procedures.

6. Melanin is essentially involved in controlling all mental and physical body activities in the MD individual. It has been shown to possess semi-conductive properties outside the body. This means that it behaves like a conductor. Sometimes it may conduct electricity. It also behaves like an insulator (just like rubber and plastic) in that melanin will not allow electrical currents to pass through its structure.

7. Melanin can bind and release most of the known elements of earth. These elements include certain minerals such as calcium, Iron, zinc, potassium, and sodium, which are essential for proper body function.

8. Melanin is present at the sight of all tissue repair and tissue regeneration. It is also present when there are infections and diseases. Melanin has a direct relationship to the immune system in MD individuals and is directly responsible for the capacity of the MD individual to resist disease. It has been found by researchers as of 1990 that synthetic melanin is one of the top-line anti-viral substances. That

is, when melanin is placed in the presence of cells and then those cells are exposed to the AIDS virus, the cells cannot be infected by the virus.

9. Melanin is capable of undergoing many chemical reactions at once through what scientists call "oxidation reduction reactions." This means that the melanin has a rhythmetric activity within its natural chemical activity. These reactions give a harmonic pattern or rhythm to the tissues in which they occur. It is felt that this is what is responsible for giving the smooth muscles of MD people their rhythm.

10. Melanin can produce or neutralize radiation and neutralize the harmful free radicals that occur from the breakdown of many food substances, and also neutralizes any harmful reactions from ultraviolet radiation.

MELANIN AND THE NERVOUS SYSTEM

Before we close our discussion on melanin, it is very important to understand its direct relationship with the nervous system. In the embryonic development of all humans, three types of germ tissues are developed, and from these three all cells evolve, forming our body.

The ectoderm (the outermost layer of germ cell tissue) contains a collection of black pigment that is crucial for the proper development of the nervous system. This black pigment in the ectoderm has been identified as melanin. That is to say, from this pigmented layer of embryonic germ tissue develop the epidermal tissues (the nails, hair, skin glands, brain, spinal cord, and external sense organs such as the ears and eyes). It is therefore obvious that melanin has a direct interaction with all nerve cell tissues and sensory organs.

The central nervous system (CNS) controls the sensory, neuromuscular and hormonal organs within the human body. Damage or malfunction of the nervous system can impair human sensitivity, movement, and consciousness. Melanin plays a dominant role in information processing that is essential for proper neurologic and metabolic function.

It is also known that melanin is necessary for proper receptivity of energy imparted to our bodies from the external environment. It is quite obvious why melanin would have a direct relationship with light. Again, we recognize that light is not just the color sensation perceived by the eye, but light is also heat, radiation, laser waves, cosmic waves, radio waves, TV waves, magnetism, and electrical currents. Due to melanin's tremendous capacity to absorb these forms of light and use them as energy sources to recharge itself and the cells in which it is located, melanin's strategic relationship with the central nervous system also gives us the capacity to immediately know what is happening to us within our external environment and to know from `where the energy exchange is coming. This gives human beings great ability to be aware of their internal environment, and to constantly be recharged and regenerated from interacting with the external environment.

It must be concluded that light, as it has been described in our previous paragraph, is a form of nutrition, especially for the MD race. More discussion of light and its nutritional factors will be discussed.

BIBLIOGRAPHY

AFRICAN PHILOSOPHY : ASSUMPTIONS AND PARADIGMS FOR RESEARCH ON BLACK PERSONS. Los Angeles: Fanon Center Publications, 1976.

BARNES, C. MELANIN: THE CHEMICAL KEY TO GREAT BLACKNESS Vol. I, Houston, TX: CB.

Knobloch, H., and Pasamick, E. FURTHER OBSERVATIONS ON THE BEHAVIORAL DEVELOPMENT OF NEGRO CHILDREN. Journal of Genetic Psychology, 83, 137-157, 1953.

Moore, K. THE DEVELOPMENTAL HUMAN. Philadelphia: W.P. Sanders, 1974.

Stewart, N.A., Ph.D. MELANIN AND SENSORY MOTOR DEVELOPMENT IN THE AFRICAN INFANT: ASSESSMENT IMPLICATIONS THESIS

Light & Health

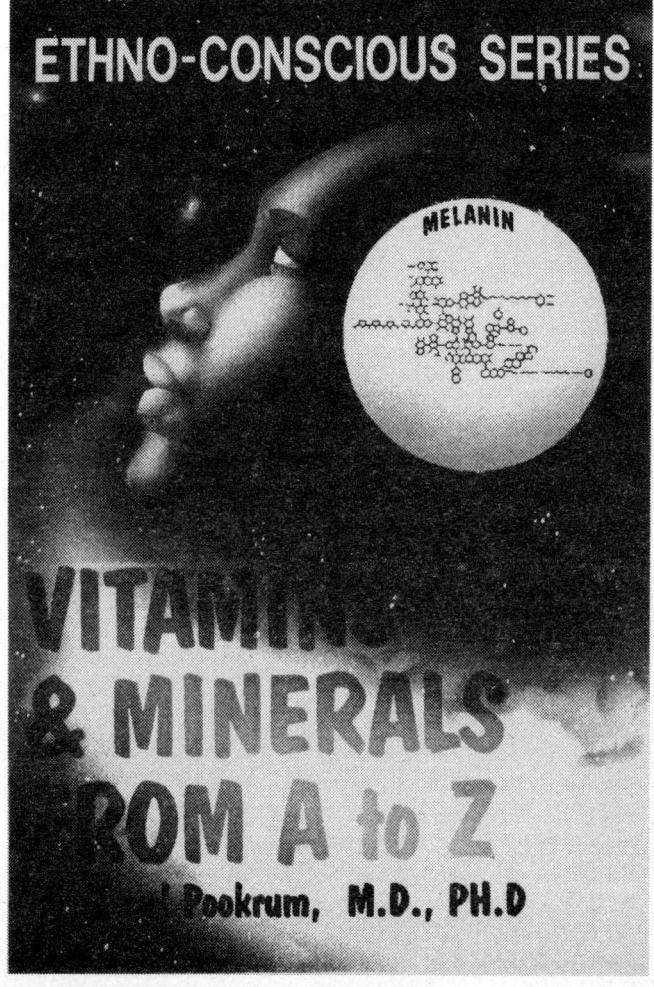

ETHNO-CONSCIOUS SERIES

MELANIN

VITAMINS & MINERALS FROM A to Z

Pookrum, M.D., PH.D

LIGHT AND HEALTH

PART I

THE PINEAL GLAND

The pineal gland resides in the center of the brain overlooking the third ventricle. It sits directly between the eyes and at a level just above the ears. It is a very mysterious gland and was named the pineal gland because it has a pine cone configuration. It is very small, about the size of a pea. For centuries it has had all kinds of mysterious and metaphysical characteristics associated with it.

The pineal gland has a direct relationship with the hypothalamus and the pituitary glands. Together, they form what was known in the Kemetic (ancient Egyptian) era as the "Sacred Triangle."

This gland exists in all animals; however, the location varies from being just under the skin and behind the head in frogs, to being in the center of the brain in humans. All pineal glands throughout all animal species, however, function the same. It is known that they are light-sensitive neuroendocrine transducers. That is, they are stimulated by light to produce hormones that are released into the blood system and through the nervous system to activate hormonal responses and metabolic regulation throughout the entire body.

In humans, there is no direct relationship between the eye and the pineal gland as there is in lower animals. Still, the uptake of light by the optic nerve is indirectly related to the pineal gland via a nerve ganglion known as the "superior cervical ganglion" located in the neck.

The pineal gland serves multiple activities in the body. Many of these activities are still not clearly understood nor identified; however, there are a few primary functions that must be discussed here. The primary function of the pineal gland in the human body is the secretion of serotonin and melatonin. These hormones are light and dark dependent. Serotonin is secreted during the daylight hours when the eye is receiving direct light. The stimulation of the optic nerve through the sympathetic nervous system to the pineal gland causes this gland to secrete serotonin. The detailed activity of serotonin in the body can be reviewed in any basic biochemistry book. Worth noting, however, is one of the main activities of serotonin is the capacity of the body to release waste from the tissues once serotonin is secreted into the blood stream.

THE PINEAL BODY

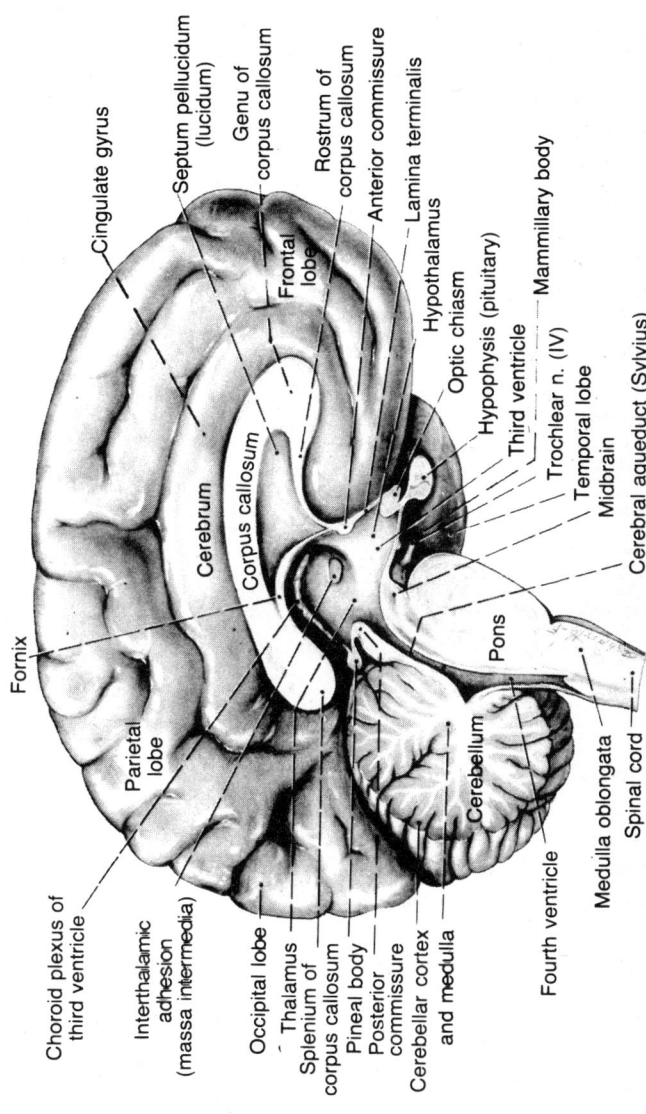

Figure 9-19. Sagittal view of the left half of the brain and spinal cord.

When the light reflected into the optic nerve has significantly diminished, the pineal gland is stimulated to begin the secretion of melatonin. Melatonin does many things. A few of its primary functions include: 1) the stimulation of the pituitary gland to secrete neurohormones that will bring about a maturity of the reproductive organs, and 2) tissue regeneration.

In summary, the pineal gland, when stimulated by light, secretes serotonin that stimulates the detoxification and waste release cycle of the body. When the gland is in the presence of darkness, it secretes melatonin, which initiates the regeneration of tissue and stimulates reproductive capacity. Melatonin also appears to be able to pass from the circulatory system into the brain and the cerebral spinal fluid without difficulty, suggesting that it may play a role in the regulation of brain function.

Humans secrete most of their melatonin at night, between 11:00 pm and 7:00 am, then stop secreting during the day. The whole sequence of events from the retina of the eye to the superior cervical ganglion to the pineal gland is controlled by the sympathetic nervous system. Light suppresses and darkness enhances nerve signals from the superior cervical ganglion to the pineal gland for melatonin synthesis and release. This daily biological rhythm is controlled by changes in the amount of external light and is abolished if the nerve track is cut, the pineal is removed, or if exposed to an unchanged amount of light.

When humans are exposed to continuous darkness, an interesting event occurs. Melatonin secretion continues to oscillate in a daily rhythm, indicating that, in addition to an external light-dark regulation cycle, there is an *internal* daily melatonin rhythm controlled by a biological clock somewhere in the brain that is linked to the pineal gland.

Melatonin is responsible for stimulating the melanocytes that contain melanosomes, which in turn contain melanin. The amount of granules in the melanosomes and the size of the melanosomes is determined by the melanocyte and the stimulation of the melanocyte by the amount of melatonin with which it comes in contact.

Please remember that the size of the melanosome determines the amount of melanin visible to the eye. When the melanosomes are large and the granules are dispersed, the skin, hair and eyes become very dark and increase their capacity to absorb light over the spectrum. When the melanosomes become quite small and the granules cluster close together, the organs containing the melanosomes appear pale or void of color, and their capacity to absorb light over the spectrum is significantly decreased.

I suspect that melanin has a direct connection to the pineal gland via the neuromelanin nerve track and that the exposure of any part of the body that is melanated to the light or darkness also contributes to the capacity of the pineal gland to function, regardless of whether the eyes are open or closed.

This brings up a very crucial point about the lifestyle activities of melanin-dominant individuals. We are now finding that exposure to radiation from color TV, exposure to abnormal wavelengths of artificial light (such as cool blue, florescent, and pink fluorescent bulbs) cause aberrant function of the pineal gland, resulting in abnormal hormonal activity initiated within the body that eventually triggers disease. Some of the primary malfunctions perpetuated in melanin-dominant individuals by persistent exposure to abnormal light frequencies are: immune deficiency disorders such as cancer, cataract formation, increased susceptibility to neurologic dysfunction, lack of motivation, and psychoneurotic diseases such as schizophrenia.

What is the relationship between light and melatonin?

Recent studies using bright artificial light have demonstrated convincingly that nocturnal melatonin secretions can be suppressed by light of sufficient intensity. Humans need more intense light to suppress melatonin than do other mammals. Studies in blind humans give variable melatonin secretion patterns. In a recent study of 10 blind people, six subjects showed an abnormal pattern of melatonin secretion, with peak melatonin production occurring at times other than at night. The remaining four subjects showed a normal melatonin profile. Serum melatonin levels in the blood are obviously influenced by the light/dark cycle to form a fundamental biological rhythm linked to seasonal variations in the day and night cycle.

The pineal gland is linked to natural and biological rhythms. Serum melatonin levels are influenced by the sleep-wake cycle and the menstrual cycle. Recent studies have shown that, with age, there is a steady decline of morning serum levels of melatonin. The prominent night time rise in serum melatonin, as seen in young people, is also markedly diminished in old age. Melatonin secretion by the pineal gland is thus flattened over time, abolishing the daily rhythm and leaving behind a rather monotone melatonin profile. It has been conjectured that menopause and the climacteric aspect of life should not be heralded as something that one should look forward to. It is a sure sign of the death of part of the brain.

It is important to remember that, to maintain healthy hormonal balance, exposing oneself to the proper natural daylight and natural night time cycles is extremely important. It is recommended that we sleep between the hours of 11 pm and 4 am, the exact times that melatonin begin to be significantly secreted from the pineal gland. Its secretions peak at 4 am and level off thereafter. The room should be completely dark, if possible, or, if light is present, it should be a blue light. We have found that the blue light is not as disruptive to the pineal gland as the onset of certain bright light upon rising, and would not abruptly diminish the hormonal activities of the pineal. So, on rising, one should remain in the sleeping room for 15-20 minutes before coming out to bright light - and if light must be in the room upon rising - it should be of a blue light frequency.

The necessary production of melatonin - and eventually its important counterpart, melanin, as in melanin-dominant individuals - is predicated on the intake of adequate B vitamins and minerals, especially calcium and magnesium. As you read further into this book, the identification of foodstuffs for these nutrients has been referenced. Please study the cross-section of the brain and commit to memory the pathway that light takes through the eye into the body.

THE VISIBLE SPECTRUM

Please study this chart very, very intently. This chart is a mathematical and pictorial demonstration of photonic vibration rate of each primary race presently on the planet earth. This chart demonstrates various spectrums of photon activity innately perceivable by each race.

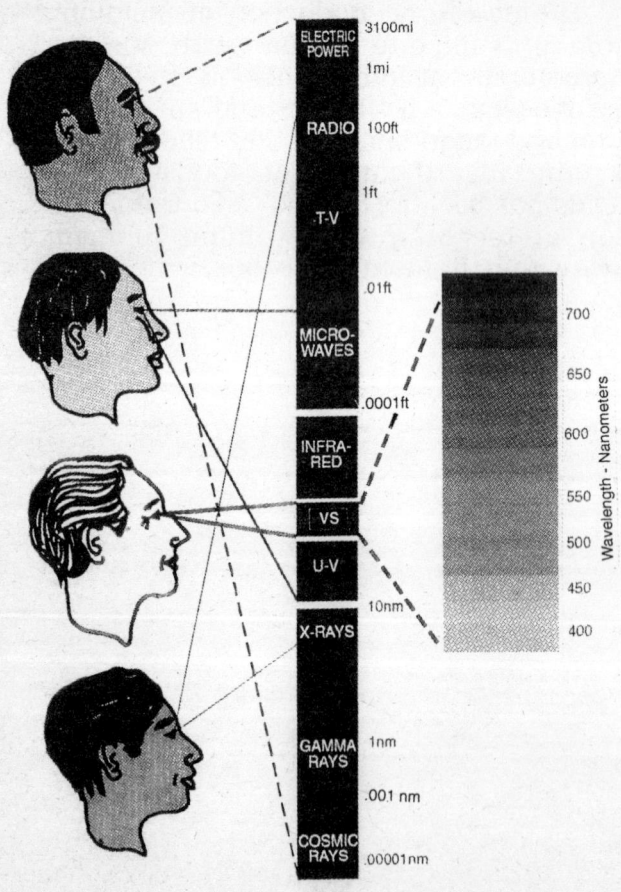

Light & Health 41

For example: The photon frequencies between 400-700 nanometers known as the "visible light" spectrum (V.S) is the standard photon movement (vibration) of the light particles composing the Causacian body. Said scientifically 400-700 nanometer is the standard photon movement of the atomic-light particles of the Caucasians electromagnetic structure. For the Caucasian to innately perceive other frequencies of light which, is synonymous to moving into another reality, would require the Caucasian to CONSCIOUSLY increase or decrease the rate of movement of the photons composing their body.

Usually this is achieved by the use of an external agent; medication, or the application of intense bombardment of their bodies with more energy, such as color, sound etc . . .

The abilities of the Caucasian to directly interact with broader range of the electromagnetic spectrum requires this race to create a transducer and or amplifying mechanism which will decrease or increase the photons within the electromagnetic spectrum moving slower or more rapidly than the visual spectrum of light(VS). The transducer or amplifying mechanism would bring into "parallel space" the photons moving more rapidly or slower than themselves with the space occupying the Perceived Visible Spectrum without losing the specific quality of the light now perceived as an "Extra" V.S. light agent. This is known as "artificial extra sensory perception".

The technologic apparatus known as Television, Radio, Microwave Ovens, etc......do this. Without these Artificial Extra Sensory Perceptive boxes", The Caucasian race would not be able to perceive these extra V.S. light frequencies which are other realities. In ancient Egyptian (African), Sanskrit (India) and Mayan (Indian) race cultures, their historic writings and pictorial records clearly indicate that they were innately aware of, interacted with, and utilized television, radio, infra-red, and x-ray frequencies within their own physical bodies, without the use of exterior mechanisms or machines.

In conclusion, if I as an African and you as a Caucasian were sitting on a scenic mountain together, enjoying a beautiful day and I as the African said to you:

"Did you hear that?"
Who's calling me?
I only told you I was coming here
today!"

The Caucasian would naturally retort:

"What are you talking about?
I didn't hear anything!
and I didn't tell anyone
We were coming here!"

Who's reality is true? Think about it!! if I have melanin which is an innate receptor of radio waves (sound waves) implanted in (12) twelve sites of my brain and as a Caucasian, having limited **Melanin (melanin recessiveness) and only two (2) sites of melanin implanted in the brain: as a Caucasian, the potential of being capable to receive and neurologically process radio waves innately is only 1/6 as great as the melanin dominant African.

Could the Caucasian equitably debate the question of "who heard what" due to the variation in their perceptive abilities?

In this example could the Caucasian discuss a reality that he may only experience less than 10% of the time in his relative awareness as a reality for someone else structurally unlike himself? The Caucasian as defined by his *melanin content and neurologic anatomical ultra-structure, experiences a reality that is only a small portion of the total reality (light perception and interaction) of the African and Indian race.

     Reality is defined here as the capacity of the body to interact with the electromagnetic spectrum.

     *It is important to remember that one's melanin content allows the individual to have prolonged exposure to and to record detail data within the DNA of one's cell: the type, intensity, and quality of electromagnetic exposure.

PART II
LIGHT

So many of us take for granted the light that permeates our environment and how it is responsible for everything that we can see, hear, feel, taste and touch, and all of the sensations of which we, as humans, are unaware.

Light consists of the following frequencies: electric waves, radio waves, infrared, shortwave infrared, red, orange, yellow, green, blue, in ultraviolet, X-ray, gamma rays, cosmic rays, and TV waves. These are all forms of light. Most of us recognize light as being the colors identifiable in the visible spectrum only - colors ranging from red to violet. However, all of the other rays listed are also considered light. We have now discovered that light is the foundation and is responsible for life.

It is important to recognize that the most important organ to receive light is the eyeball. This is a very, very important form of nutrition. Our eyes use their basic nutritional food (light) to bring about health. Inadequate light brings disease to the physical body. Since vision is truly our navigational system, taking in more information per unit of time and from a broader area of space than any of our other senses, it is useful to examine how our eyes use light to accomplish this task.

Each eye contains 137 million photo receptors. There are approximately 130 million photoreceptors called rods, and 75 million called cones. Cones, which function primarily in daylight, are concerned with visual acuity and color discrimination at high intensity of illumination. Rods, which function primarily in twilight and at night, are mostly concerned with colorless vision and movement at low levels of illumination. The rods are also responsible for the relay of information concerning the non-visible spectrum of light. The rods inform the brain and body about the amount of X-ray, radio waves, TV waves, infrared, electric, cosmic, gamma and ultraviolet waves to which the body is exposed.

This level of perception via the rods of the eyes is directly independent upon the amount of melanin or pigment in the rods. The pigment in the rods is known as "rodopsin." Eyes that are pale in color - ranging from pink (in individuals suffering from albinism) to all ranges of hazel eyes, have a defect in their capacity to perceive complete information regarding the non-visible light they are receiving. The darker the eye, the more accurately the body is able to perceive the intensity and the degree of exposure to non-visible light spectrum activity. It is also interesting to note that individuals with darker eyes and more pigment in the rods also have the built-in capacity to tolerate more of the non-visible spectrum. They are capable of receiving information via the rods through the sympathetic nervous system to the pineal gland, hypothalamus, pituitary glands, and other areas of the brain, such as the limbic system and the corpus calossum. This allows their bodies to respond differently in time and space based on this additional information. It has been identified that individuals with melanin in the eye have a greater capacity to know of the existence of other objects and information than do individuals who do not have melanated photoreceptivity within the eye.

A very good example is the Dogon tribe in West Africa. Because they contain concentrated amounts of melanin, they are capable of receiving radio waves from star systems, especially the Dog Star, Sirius, and have recorded its movements throughout the history of their tribe, using its celestial configurations to decorate garments, vessels, houses and living quarters within the tribe, even though they lack radio telescopes to optically "see" this star system.

The photoreceptors of the eye transform light into electrical impulses that are then sent to the brain at approximately 234 miles per hour. These impulses travel along several different routes that involve the entire brain. Some travel to the visual cortex for the construction of images, while others travel to the brain's hypothalamus and affect our vital functions. Although vision is perhaps our most dynamic process, constantly changing in accordance with our mental and physical state, most of us think of the eyes as having only a single function: eyesight. We are not aware that eyesight is merely a small aspect of that dynamic process known as vision.

We are much less aware that our eyes are the major access routes by which light enters the body. They can be mirrors of our general and emotional health, as well as accurate indicators of our styles of thinking and learning. This is extremely important, since this ancient, yet newly discovered, connection between the eye and brain function is the link that binds us with nature.

It was not until the early 1970s that science was able to prove that light entering the eye was not just for purposes of vision, but was also being sent to one of the most important parts of the brain: the hypothalamus. Light entering the eye serves both visual and non-visual functions. It is interesting to note that ancient civilizations were quite aware of this, and in their oral traditions and limited written texts, always taught both levels of vision. When we speak about health, balance, and physiological regulation, we are referring to the functions of the body's major health keepers: the nervous system and the endocrine system. These major control systems of the body are directly stimulated and regulated by light.

In summary, light enters the eyes not only to serve vision, but to go directly to the body's biological clock within the hypothalamus. The hypothalamus controls the nervous system and endocrine system, whose combined effect regulates all biological functions in humans. In addition, the hypothalamus controls most of the body's regulatory functions by monitoring light-related information and sending it to the pineal, which then uses this information to cue other organs about light conditions in the environment.

The study of color in the Western World has been undertaken for hundreds of years, and the papers and research regarding color and the entire light spectrum has produced mounds and mounds of information. I ask my readers to begin to investigate the multitude of books that have been written on color and light. I suggest this research to stimulate the question as to how their lifestyle may create a condition known as *malillumination*.

In recent times, we have become aware that we are constantly ingesting polluted air and devitalized food. Yet, the most obvious nutrient, light, has been overlooked. Just as an improper diet may cause malnutrition so an improper light diet may cause malillumination, which has severe adverse effects upon health. Light is a major nutrient sustaining all life; therefore, poor or incomplete lighting will significantly affect every aspect of human existence. This is extremely important for the melanin-dominant individual, in that melanin production, hormonal regulation and balance, immune system activity, and many other necessary physiologic activities in melanin-dominant individuals are all predicated on light and dark exposure. Inappropriate light exposure or exposure to artificial sources of light have been identified as being very dangerous to humans.

Malillumination is a crucial factor in the health of melanin-dominant individuals, especially melanin-dominant individuals living in urban areas where cement buildings and artificial lighting interfere with the absorption of full spectrum light and also expose melanin-dominant individuals to abnormal light sources.

In considering the role light plays in influencing health, it is important to first look at the constituents of sunlight as well as the kinds of artificial light to which we are exposed in our daily lives.

Light is composed of waves of radiant energy. It is measured in wavelengths, the distances between two consecutive rests. Visible light ranges from 400 to 700 nanometers in wavelength. Gamma rays, X-rays, and ultraviolet rays have wavelengths shorter than 400 nanometers; infrared light, microwave, and radio wave have wavelengths longer than 700 nanometers. Sunlight, which contains ALL the different wavelengths, provides the total electromagnetic spectrum (light) under which all life on this planet has evolved and to which it must be exposed.

Thomas Edison and associates' invention of the incandescent light bulb was a quantum leap in technology. It simultaneously created a situation in which people lost respect for nature's daily light-dark cycle and began burning the candle at both ends. With the growing availability of the light bulb, life became largely an indoor event, drastically reducing the amount of time to which people exposed themselves to full spectrum light. Please study the electromagnetic spectrum chart on page .40..

Let us look at a few of the problems that inappropriate exposure to light can create. It has been discovered that exposure to certain frequencies of light affect muscle tone and strength of the shoulder girdle. An experiment done in December

1978 at one of the larger research hospitals in the United States disclosed the following:

Modest amounts of near ultraviolet light as part of a visually balanced solar-like spectrum increased shoulder muscle tone and improved short-term strength compared to warm, white fluorescent lights of comparable illumination.

Radio frequencies in the 0.1-100 megahertz range also appeared to weaken shoulder girdle strength.

Specific exclusion of near ultraviolet as is common with usual fluorescent and incandescent lights, reduced muscle tone and strength. The time constant (time to observe the effect) appeared to be 3-6 seconds.

Proper shielding of radio frequencies restored muscle tone and strength.

Red dominant illumination weakens more than blue dominant illumination. Radiation from digital watches is within governmental safety levels; however, it grossly weakens the muscles of the arm. Sun glasses, including those that darken when worn in sunlight, and ordinary eye glasses that block the ultraviolet cause measurable loss of muscle strength.

It has also been identified that Pyrex glass, due to the type of electromagnetic frequency that it emits and attracts from the body, when held in the hand also causes muscle weakness in the upper part of the body. It would be very interesting to measure the amount of life force energy remaining in food that is cooked in Pyrex cookware.

It is important to know that there is a phenomenon known as biological combustion. This is a natural phenomenon that occurs in the physical body relative to the specific wavelength frequencies of the individual to absorb nutrients. Biological combustion must occur in all nutritional activity, including that involving medicine. All nutritional substances, including drugs, have a specific wavelength absorption. If those wavelengths are missing in the artificial light source a person is exposed to, no biological combustion will take place, and the nutritional benefits of the particular substance will not be utilized. In other words, if the light carrying capacity within your body is not equal to the wavelength frequency of the foods you eat, you will not have, the capacity to combust that food completely and absorb its nutrients, which are also light force. So, when we talk about nutrition from an atomic standpoint, we are talking about the absorption and emission of wavelengths of light.

As melanin-dominant individuals, it is very important to realize that we must be exposed to the entire electromagnetic spectrum. We do require ultraviolet radiation for health. We have found, however, that ultraviolet radiation can be harmful for those individuals who are melanin-recessive. Plants, animals and humans who are melanin-dominant do require ultraviolet radiation for maximum activity and stimulation of the hormonal system and metabolism. The use of sun glasses, tinted lens glasses, tinted contact lenses, eyeglasses and contact lenses that are not made from full spectrum material that is, special transparent materials that will - allow the full spectrum of light and ultraviolet to pass through it - is quite harmful for the melanin-dominant individual. Numerous studies have revealed to us the importance of ultraviolet radiation in the pigmented world of life. Plants, animals and melanin-dominant individuals require this.

In regard to the hole in the ozone layer, melanin-dominant individuals who are free of food toxins, who are not drug dependent, and who are capable of receiving adequate amounts of fresh air and water, will be able to make enough melanin to counteract the dangerous concentrations of ultraviolet radiation that may be emitted. The concern that melanin-recessive individuals have is that they do not make melanin in any amounts sufficient to protect them from the ultraviolet radiation of normal filtered sunlight. Therefore, the hole in the ozone layer, which has lost its natural filter due to hydrocarbon combustion, is a real threat for individuals who are melanin-recessive. Fair-skinned melanin-dominant individuals are also at risk for genetic damage and metabolic disorders due to the limited amount of melanin. I recommend that melanin-dominant individuals who are considered fair-skinned use sun blockers with at least a sun screen factor of three when outdoors. Melanin-dominant individuals who are gold-brown, red-brown, brown, black to blue-black are protected. The gold-brown and red-brown individuals, however, should expose themselves to full spectrum light for longer periods of time during the day to begin to stimulate more melanin activity so that as the ultraviolet radiation increases, the body will be lined with adequate amounts of protective melanin, and it will not harm the nuclei of their cells or destroy the epithelia layers of their skin.

In summary, light is one of the most important nutrients for melanin-dominant individuals. Full-spectrum light - including X-rays, cosmic rays, radio waves, TV waves, radiant heat, long ultra-violet rays - are important for the health of melanin-dominant individuals. It is recommended that a thorough study of light and its phenomenon and effect upon human life be undertaken by melanin-dominant individuals and become part of the educational system in all schools with a predominant melanin-dominant student population.

WAYS TO PREVENT MALILLUMINATION

A.   Windows, sliding doors, and skylights. Identify the types that your home or environment contains. There are at least two commercial brands of ultraviolet-transmitting plastic available. One is UVT Acrylite, manufactured by the American Cyanamide; the other is UVT Plexiglass, manufactured by the Rohm and Haas Company. Both companies also make ultraviolet absorbing plastics that do not transmit the ultraviolet, so it is important to be sure to get the UVT plastic, not the UVA. The plastic comes with a protective paper covering that should show exactly what type it is. It also comes in various thicknesses. It is advisable to use as thin a piece as possible for two reasons: 1) the thinner it is, the more ultraviolet will penetrate it, and 2) the thicker it is, the more it costs.

For those of you who are not aware of the qualities of plastic, please note that plastic possesses much better insulating qualities than does glass, and when plastic windows 1/8" thick are installed, there is no need for storm windows. In washing these windows, use a sponge or chamois with soap and water. Plastic does not scratch easily. Do not use chemical cleaners containing ammonia or other chemicals.

B.   Eyeglasses. Ultraviolet-transmitting spectacle lenses are manufactured by Armor Light Inc. as "full spectrum" lenses, and by Eye Craft Optical, Inc. as "sunlight lenses." These are available in clear or neutral gray for sun glasses if necessary. Bausch and Lomb soft lens "contact lenses" are also ultraviolet-transmitting. Ask for them whenever you get your glasses. Note that individuals who have had operations for cataracts should not wear contact lenses. It has been reported that decreased oxygen content to the eye due to microvascular atherosclerosis or significant and chronic B-vitamin deficiencies (especially of glutathione), and malillumination are the main reasons for cataract formation. Cataract formation is quite common in melanin-dominant individuals living above the 42nd degree latitude, which makes them prime candidates for malillumination, and also in individuals who eat diets high in saturated fats (animal products and byproducts), which directly contributes to microvascular atherosclerosis.

C.   Fluorescent lights. All fluorescent tubes give off radiation that should be shielded, so it is necessary to use lighting fixtures that provide this. Full-spectrum radiation, shielded fluorescent fixtures are currently being manufactured by Acme Dunbar Industries, Inc., 1130 West Cornelia St., Chicago, IL. These fixtures also provide a separate socket for the black light ultraviolet fluorescent tube so that it may be replaced as needed. This is necessary because the phosphorus that gives off the ultraviolet wavelength has a burning life of only 7,000-9,000 hours, whereas the visible phosphorus will last up to 36,000 hours.

D.   Colors for interior decorating. The wavelengths of light reflected from a colored surface behave in the same way as wavelengths passing through a colored filter. The only difference is that the color filter transmits certain wavelengths and blocks or stops others. The colored surface reflects certain wavelengths and absorbs others. The end results are the same as far as the wavelengths that reach the eye or surface of the skin are concerned. Therefore, in keeping with the full-spectrum theory, a room should not be all one color and preferably not even all the walls one strong color, especially not pink or orange. White is the exception, as white reflects all colors or wavelengths. However, some white substances reflect more ultraviolet than others. It is recommended that colors for ceilings and walls be white or light pastel shades of blue, green, gray or beige. Accent with other colors even small spots of pink and orange in the curtains, furniture and floor-covering. make it as much as possible like the natural colors indoor. Remember, the brilliant pinks and oranges of sunset last only about 15 minutes, which has been determined as the maximum time a person can be left in the pink cell of correctional centers in prisons before the beneficial short term effects begin to give way to the long term effects of increased depression, aggression, and violence.

E. Television sets and video display terminals. A long standing problem - and potentially lethal problem of televisions and video display terminals - has been the amount of radiation that these instruments emit. There have been many attempts to try to correct this, from repositioning the tube in the box to lead cabinets. It is recommended that TV cabinets be shielded with lead and that one should sit at least 15 feet from color televisions.

It is impossible to sit 15 feet away from video display terminals in that one needs to be very close to them in order to enter data into the computer. However, lead screens that go over the front of the display unit help to diminish the amount of radiation. Another option is to have a fadeout screen, on which, when one is not actually working at the computer, will diminish the amount of light passing through the cathode until one is ready to enter data into the computer. Software is available that shuts down the screen with a selectable period of time after cessation of data entry into the computer. A touch of any key will re-activate the screen. Remember, a TV picture tube or video terminal display tube is a cathode ray tube and works on the same principle as an X-ray tube. Several companies are considering using basic mirrors as reflectors of the information from the screen so that one does not have to sit directly in front of the screen to see the image. It is important to remember to keep children a minimum of 15 feet away from TV sets and to sit level with the TV, as opposed to lying underneath it where most of the radiation is projected.

For further enlightenment regarding the full-light spectrum, a 46-minute color and sound film may be purchased from International Film Bureau, 332 S. Michigan Avenue, Chicago, IL 60604, (313) 427-4545. This film is quite educational regarding full-spectrum light, its advantages and side-effects.

SUGGESTIONS FOR OUTDOOR LIVING

It has been identified that smoke detectors, digital watches, and synthetic materials all interfere with the absorption of full spectrum light. Therefore, it is recommended that these items not be included in the environment or that they are put in a safe place that is not the sleeping and living quarters of the home. In order to obtain the maximum benefits from living outdoors under natural conditions, a minimum of six hours a day of natural daylight is suggested. For people living in large cities, this may be rather difficult, but it is hoped the following suggestions may be helpful:

Bringing in artificial light for sitting indoors, and looking through ordinary windows or windshield glass should be avoided.

Wearing of ordinary glasses, particularly dark glasses, should be avoided.

Ultraviolet-transmitting spectacles and windows that let natural daylight come indoors are recommended; sleeping outdoors as much as possible on a screened porch in the spring and summer is recommended.

The glandular system is more sensitive to light immediately following the night sleep . In particular, artificial light sources and sunlight filtered through glass should be avoided, even for brief periods of a few moments during the first hour or two after awakening in the morning, or following any rest during the daytime. For this reason, a dim blue night light, such as a Christmas tree ornament light should be used so as not to interrupt the night with ordinary electrical lights, which seem particularly bright when the eyes are accustomed to total darkness.

If it is necessary to remain indoors, ordinary glass windows should be kept open as much as possible and curtains drawn across any portion of glass that will not be open.

If a person is being driven in an automobile, it is best to look out through the open side windows rather than through the windshield ahead. Constant interruption of the natural sunlight by either artificial light or sunlight filtered through glass, even for brief periods, can offset the benefits received from light exposure and should be consciously avoided.

It is not necessary to be in full, direct sunlight, and for those persons who are melanin-recessive, direct sunlight should be avoided. However, for melanin-dominant persons, direct sunlight is not a problem if one is accustomed to being outdoors. For those individuals who are melanin-dominant and are not accustomed to being outdoors, one should ease oneself into the presence of direct sunlight. Exposure for only 20 minutes a day for two days is recommended prior to exposure longer than 20 minutes. After the first two days, sun exposure may be increased up to two hours daily or more. Initially, avoid sunbathing between the hours of 11:00 a.m. and 3:00 p.m. After the initial 48 hours of limited sun exposure, the best hours to sunbathe are 10:00 a.m. - 12:00 noon and 2:00 p.m. - 4:00 p.m for melanin-dominant people.

Vitamins

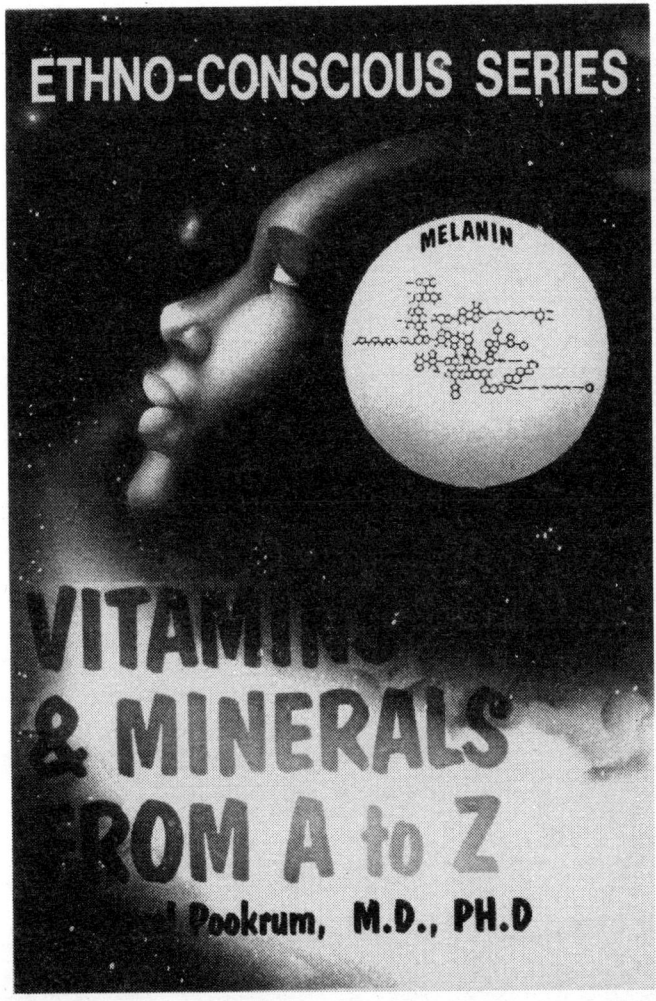

VITAMINS

VITAMIN A (BETA CAROTENE)

Vitamin A prevents night blindness and other eye problems. It also supports healthy skin and can be an aid to preventing acne. Vitamin A enhances immunity, helps to heal and prevent gastro-intestinal ulcers, protects against pollution and cancer formation, and is needed for tissue and skin repair. It assists in the formation of bones and teeth and aids in the storage of fat. Vitamin A protects against colds,[6] influenza and infections. This vitamin acts as an antioxidant that helps protect the cells against deterioration, cancer, and other metabolic malfunction diseases. Note that Vitamin A slows the aging process. ·Note further that protein cannot be properly utilized without this supplement.

In man, foods containing beta carotene are converted to Vitamin A in the liver. The Eskimos, who are nearly 100% flesh eaters require Vitamin A and use the polar bear as a source. However they have an ancient process to extract Vitamin from liver so it will not be too toxic to the human system. Therefore, we should be very careful when eating polar bear livers. (Smile) For the melanin dominant individual,

---

[6] Iron should be taken separately, but may be omitted if no deficiency exists. Do not take in multisupplement formula.

the natural source of Vitamin A should be from plant origin.

Sources

Vitamin A can be found in green and yellow fruits and vegetables. Foods containing significant amounts include: alfalfa, apricots, asparagus, beets, broccoli, cantaloupe, carrots, Swiss chard (be careful eating this if you have kidney stones, gall stones, bladder problems, kidney conditions or acid skin reaction), dandelion greens, garlic, kale, mustard, papaya, parsley, peaches, red peppers, spirulina, pumpkin, yellow squash, turnip greens and watercress.

Warning

Vitamin A should not be taken in large amounts in pill form or as cod liver oil by those suffering from liver disease. Pregnant women should not take amounts of Vitamin A over 25,000 International Units (IU). Children should be given only very low doses of Vitamin A, and melanin-dominant individuals should ensure that they eat food sources of Vitamin A all year round.

Antibiotics, laxatives and some cholesterol lowering drugs interfere with Vitamin A absorption. If you have been taking antibiotics for any reason and for any length of time, you may be creating the foundation for Vitamin A deficiency. So watch your diet. Antibiotics have become an extremely dangerous drug and one should investigate one's diet and herb sources to treat infectious states in the body before taking antibiotic therapy. Antibiotics should be used as a last resort measure because of the TREMENDOUS side effects they activate.

Diabetics should avoid large amounts of beta carotene, as should hypothyroid individuals, because they cannot easily convert beta carotene to Vitamin A.

NOTE: Do a little research for yourself. What is the name of true Vitamin A, that is, the form of Vitamin A your liver produces? Remember that beta carotene is the precursor of Vitamin A and that the liver actually makes Vitamin A. So please recognize that this is another vitamin that our body will make for itself if given the proper building blocks.

VITAMIN C (ASCORBIC ACID)

Vitamin C is an antioxidant required for tissue growth and repair. This antioxidant is required for tissue growth and repair, adrenal gland function, and healthy gums. Vitamin C protects against the harmful effects of pollution, against cancer and infection, and enhances immunity. It also assists in reducing cholesterol levels and high blood pressure, thus helping to prevent atherosclerosis. Vitamin C is essential in the formation of collagen (see dictionary). Furthermore, it protects against blood clotting and promotes the healing and production of anti-stress hormones. It also aids in interferon production. This vitamin is also needed for the metabolism of folic acid, tyrosine and thiamine. All of these amino acids are discussed later.

New evidence indicates that Vitamin C and Vitamin E work synergistically. Vitamin E scavenges for dangerous oxygen radicals in the cell membrane while Vitamin C breaks down free radicals in biologic fluids. Together, these vitamins greatly extend antioxidant activity.

A New Breakthrough

"Ester C. Polyascorbate" is a breakthrough in the use of Vitamin C, especially for those suffering from chronic illness due to cancer and AIDS. This form of Vitamin C, which is an esterified form, was first researched by Jonathan Wright, M.D. Dr. Wright proved that white blood cell ascorbate levels increased four times more with Ester Vitamin C than with ordinary Vitamin C or ascorbic Acid, and only one-third of the amount is excreted through the urine! Vitamin C is normally a water soluble vitamin, that is, not bound to protein or retained for use by the cell. It is excreted in the urine.

The feeling in the health profession for years was that Vitamin C could not be manufactured by the body. However, such authors as Michio Kushi of the East-West Foundation (Boston, MA) states that Vitamin C IS MADE IN THE ADRENAL GLANDS in small amounts, depending on the diet and the individual's environmental location. If an individual takes in large amounts of Vitamin C, the cells in the adrenal glands will not manufacture Vitamin C spontaneously because the "feedback mechanism" of the body will not stimulate its production. Therefore, minimum amounts of Vitamin C must remain in the bloodstream to activate and maintain activation of the Vitamin C-producing cells.

I feel this is a more ideal situation because the ability always to have Vitamin C on board is present when we do not overload our bodies with the vitamin from exogenous sources.

Sources

It has been noted that in tropical environments, many of the plants normally carry high amounts of Vitamin C. This characteristic of plants makes the environment conducive for man because of the role Vitamin C plays in stimulating immune system function. In tropical climates, there are many, many insects and many breeding organisms that could possibly attack the human body and bring about disease. So nature prepares us to deal with what it has created in her total environment by providing foods for us that will keep us healthy, if we will only eat what is provided in that environment and also maintain the proper state of mind and spirit.

Those of us who live in the temperate zone are also provided with natural sources of Vitamin C for use when necessary. How does this work? When the temperature increases during our spring and summer months, nature provides foods that are high in Vitamin C, such as green leafy vegetables and our spring berries (strawberries and raspberries). Then it provides our summer fruits that are high in Vitamin C: cherries, plums, pears, summer apples, and, finally, melons.

In the wintertime, the threat of bug and bacterial infestation is reduced due to the typically cold weather. Insect eggs are in dormancy or have died. The chance for infections is significantly reduced. Correspondingly for this time of year, the natural production of Vitamin C-bearing plants is reduced in the food chain. Consequently, our Vitamin C intake in the winter should be minimal, while the production of this vitamin in our adrenal glands should increase sufficiently to keep the immune system stimulated for warding off any type of infectious organisms present in the environment.

I feel it is quite dangerous to take large quantities of Vitamin C all year long, mainly because at some point one actually burns out the immune system. The immune system is tricked into unnecessary activity with the ingestion of high dosages of Vitamin C. Indeed, the immune system always wants to stay alert, but the false stimulation for defense against full-blown disease is a different story.

I suspect that the immune system of most individuals in the United States and other Western countries is very poor because of either over-stimulation from food and/or vitamin supplement abuse. Food abuse occurs when people in temperate zones eat tropical fruit all year round. This is a no-no! Tropical fruit should be eaten only in the tropics or as a dietary variation while in the temperate zone, but only once or twice a year no more. People who take street drugs and pharmaceutical drugs, for whatever reason, also are among those who are stimulating (and finally depressing) immune system activity. So, we must be very, very careful about recognizing that we need more or less of certain vitamins, depending upon the living environment, the work environment, and our daily choice of activity.

Before closing, let us go back to Ester C. It enters the blood stream four times quicker and into the blood cells more efficiently. This is a big step for the immune system. Ester C has naturally chelated (bonded) minerals that allow for rapid absorption. The mineral forms include calcium, magnesium, potassium, zinc and sodium. These z pH balance forms are manufactured according to specifications.

As for additional sources of Vitamin C from those discussed earlier, they include green vegetables, citrus fruits, asparagus, avocados, broccoli, Brussels sprouts, collard greens, grapefruit, mangos, lemons, mustard greens, onions, oranges, papaya, parsley, green peas, peppers, persimmons, pineapples, radishes, rose hips (the main wintertime source for Native Americans in the temperate environment), spinach (watch out for your kidneys when eating spinach), Swiss chard (high acidity can affect the skin), tomatoes (not to be trusted), turnip greens, and watercress.

Warning

Aspirin, alcohol, analgesics, antidepressants, anticoagulants, oral contraceptives and steroids may reduce levels of Vitamin C in the body. A drug known as "diabinase" and sulfur drugs may not be effective when taking Vitamin C. Please remember that taking large doses of Vitamin C may cause a false negative reading when testing your stools for blood. That is to say that if you are taking high amounts of Vitamin C and your doctor's test of your stool for blood is positive, PLEASE inform the doctor about the vitamins. Otherwise, he/she may suspect rectal cancer and will put you through a lot of unnecessary tests. The key for you is to be assertive; speak up. Remember how vitamins and minerals can affect your body. For example, pregnant women should use amounts no larger than 5,000 mg of Vitamin C per day. Infants may become dependent upon this supplement and develop scurvy. The best food for babies during the pregnancy comes from the mother's balanced diet. After the baby is born, the mother's breast milk provides the needed nutrients.

VITAMIN D

Vitamin D is required for calcium and phosphate absorption and utilization. It is necessary for growth generally, and especially for normal growth and development of bones and teeth in children. It is important for the prevention and treatment of osteoporosis and hypocalcium, and enhances immunity. The Vitamin D that we get from food or supplements is meant to be a reactivator. It requires conversion by the liver and by the kidney before it becomes fully active. People with liver or kidney disorders are at a higher risk for osteoporosis.

The sun's ultraviolet rays can be converted directly into Vitamin D. Exposing the face and arms three times a week is effective. This is an important source of Vitamin D for melanin-dominant individuals. People with melanin can, just by being out in the sun for approximately 20 minutes two to three times weekly, produce within the skin all of the Vitamin D they need. From our previous discussion on ethnicity relative to minerals and vitamins, melanin-dominant persons have a larger bone mass than those of the Caucasian race, and thus have a greater need for larger amounts of calcium. It is quite in line that melanin-dominant persons would be created with a natural means to have the precursor necessary to metabolize calcium. That natural means of acquiring Vitamin D is right in the skin. So, after sunbathing, melanin-dominant people are not to water bathe for approximately 20 minutes. Why? with the Vitamin D made on the surface of the skin, you will want time for the skin to absorb it and take it into the blood stream. It appears Caucasians have a problem with acquiring Vitamin D because they are melanin-deficient. Constant exposure to the sun for them can be lethal through the creation of skin cancers, leathery skin, et. They must rely on exogenous sources of Vitamin D.

Sources

Natural sources of Vitamin D can be found in the skin of melanin-dominant individuals after sun exposure, as well as in fish liver oils, fatty saltwater fish, and dairy products fortified with Vitamin D. Melanin-dominant races should not eat dairy products. It has been found that 80% of the melanin-dominant races throughout the world are dairy and milk intolerant after age 5. Eating dairy products will set down a foundation for blockage diseases in the melanin-dominant body. Eggs contain Vitamin D. The vitamin is also found in alfalfa, butter, cod liver oil, egg yolk, halibut, liver, oatmeal, sweet potatoes and vegetable oils.

Warning

Toxicity may occur when amounts ingested exceed 65,000 international units (IU) over a period of years. Vitamin D should not be taken without calcium. Intestinal disorders in liver, and gall bladder malfunction interfere with absorption of Vitamin D. How can you tell if you have sluggish liver and gall bladder? You have a bad temperament, are angry and upset all the time, holler and scream often.

You can look at your face, too. See if you have circles and moles on your face, especially on the temples and the areas lateral to the jaw. You must be careful about taking additional vitamins that have Vitamin D, especially if you are melanin-dominant. You should beware of taking in too much Vitamin D because you already have it in your skin. The use of some cholesterol lowering drugs such as antacids, mineral oils and steroid hormones (e.g., cortisone) interfere with Vitamin D absorption. Thiazide diuretics disturb the calcium/Vitamin D ratio. If you are hypertensive, look up the name of the medication you are taking. If it is a thiazide diuretic, or if it contains thiazide, you need to be advised on how to obtain proper Vitamin D and proper calcium. REMEMBER: If you are melanin-dominant, you must look to your diet. Oatmeal, vegetable oils, and especially alfalfa, are a source of Vitamin D. The sunshine on your skin will always make Vitamin D for you!

VITAMIN E

Vitamin E is an antioxidant. Vitamin E prevents cancer and cardiovascular disease with the proper mental and spiritual status. This supplement improves circulation, repairs tissue and is useful in treating fibrocystic breast and premenstrual syndrome.

At this point I will interject that premenstrual syndrome and fibrocystic disease, as women associated diseases, are also an indication that there is an emotional disturbance around the concept of being female. Further, fibrocystic breast is a blockage disease of the lymphatic ducts of the breasts. The blockage is usually created by eating caffeine, chocolate, yogurt, and other dairy products. This is especially true for the melanin-dominant race. Caucasian race are much more tolerant of dairy products and can more easily eliminate these products from their system. Women who suffer from premenstrual syndrome also usually suffer from sugar addiction in some form, and therefore usually also suffer from Vitamin E deficiency.

Vitamin E promotes normal clotting and healing (thereby reducing scarring from many types of wounds), reduces blood pressure, aids in preventing cataracts, improves athletic performance, and aids in easing leg cramps. Vitamin E also prevents cell damage by inhibiting liquid "peroxidation" and by forming free radicals. It retards aging and may prevent age spots as well. I recognize age spots as another sign of blockage disease. These spots are typically referred to as freckles or moles that occur down the neck, on the breasts, all over the face, on the back of the hands, etc.

The body needs zinc in order to maintain a proper level of Vitamin E in the blood. This relationship is another example of synergy.

Sources

Vitamin E is found in the following sources: cold pressed vegetable oils, whole grains, dark green leafy vegetables, nuts, seeds, and legumes. Significant quantities of this vitamin are also found in dried beans, cornmeal, eggs, oatmeal, sweet potatoes and wheat germ. Again, by eating from the basic food table and using the proper oils, you will be able to pick up the correct amount of Vitamin E.

Warning

Do not take Iron supplements at the same time you take Vitamin E. Those suffering from diabetes, rheumatic heart disease, or an overactive thyroid should not use high doses. Those suffering from high blood pressure should start with a small amount and increase slowly to the desired amount.

VITAMIN K

Vitamin K is needed for blood clotting. It may also prevent osteoporosis. This vitamin converts glucose into glycogen for storage in the liver. Vitamin K is a very interesting vitamin. You do not need a lot of it. Vitamin K, in combination with other prenatal vitamins, figures significantly in birth defects. So, prenatal vitamins could be a hazard, causing problems when too much Vitamin D and/or two much Vitamin K are present. For this reason, eating a well balanced diet while pregnant is preferable to relying on a vitamin supplement. When vitamin supplements are needed in pregnancy due to an inability to eat a well balanced diet (or the lack of desire to eat), please get a vitamin supplement that has a minimum RDA rating. Do not purchase the high-potency augmented vitamins. The baby might be born with problems.

Sources

Vitamin K is found in alfalfa. Have you noticed that alfalfa has been mentioned as a source in almost all the vitamins? And who eats alfalfa? Cows! And they do great things with their bodies, as you may notice. For human beings, especially as melanin-dominant humans, the plant world is our best friend, and we need to be aware of what parts we need to eat. Alfalfa sprouts are excellent sources of the vitamins needed for melanin-dominant individuals, and do not cause blockage diseases that have a tendency to occur from ingesting dairy products and eating flesh. Additional sources are: broccoli, dark green leafy vegetables, soybeans, and blackstrap molasses (which is very high in minerals).

Others sources include Brussels sprouts, green leafy cabbage (the only suitable type unless it is eaten in winter), cauliflower, oatmeal, whole oats, whole rye, sunflower oil, and wheat. Please be careful in your use of oats. It is better to eat steel-cut oats or whole oat groats than to eat ordinary oatmeal on a regular basis, particularly if you have a mucus production problem. Please do some research on the processing of whole grains to determine what steel-cut oats are versus whole oat groats. Go to the natural food store and ask for either or both. Identify them by eye and then you can see the difference. They should taste different, too.

Warning

When synthetic Vitamin K is used in large doses during the last weeks of pregnancy, it may result in a toxic reaction in the newborn. Megadoses can accumulate and cause flushing and sweating. Antibiotics can interfere with the absorption of Vitamin K. Therefore, if you have been taking large amounts of antibiotics for whatever reason (acne can be one), know that you are Vitamin K deficient. Please consult the source list and get busy eating those foods to replace Vitamin K. Check with a nutritionist to discover what you can do with foods and herbs to circumvent taking antibiotics. Antibiotics have caused many problems, and we are in a dangerous state of disequilibrium because of antibiotics. Unless they are absolutely necessary to sustain life, avoid antibiotics.

VITAMIN B

Vitamin B-Complex

The B vitamins help to maintain healthy nerves, skin, eyes, hair, liver and mouth, as well as muscle tone in the digestive tract. B+ vitamins are "coenzymes" involved in energy production, and may be useful for depression or anxiety. The B vitamins should always be taken together, because they function as a team. Note that up two or three times more B vitamins can be taken for a disorder than can other vitamins.

Vitamin B_1 (Thiamine)

Thiamine enhances circulation and assists in the production of hydrochloric acid. It is also important in blood formation and carbohydrate metabolism. Thiamine affects growth disorders and learning capacity and is used for normal muscle tone for the intestines, stomach and heart. It is extremely important in the digestion process. If an insufficient quality of hydrochloric acid is produced in the walls of the stomach, protein will not be adequately broken down. This incomplete protein breakdown will result in problems such as gas and very foul-smelling bowel movements. Moles may appear on the skin because the protein is not being completely digested and eliminated through the lymphatic system. Lack of proper production of hydrochloric acid can also be the cause of an increased number of bacteria in the stomach, leading to halitosis (bad breath).

Sources

The food sources are foreign and crude: dried beans, brown rice, peanuts, peas, rice bran, soybeans, wheat germ and whole grains, asparagus, broccoli, Brussel sprouts, most nuts, oatmeal, plums, dried prunes and raisins.

Warning

Antibiotics, sulfur drugs and oral contraceptives may decrease thiamine levels in the body. A high carbohydrate diet increases the need for thiamine. Beriberi, a nervous system disease is caused by thiamine deficiency. For those of you who are quite nervous and irritable, who find that you are losing your strength, losing your grip, and/or whose feet burn, fingertips burn, experience numbness in the hands or feet check out your B vitamins and your sources of thiamine. You will probably feel much better by increasing your food sources of this vitamin.

VITAMIN B_2 (RIBOFLAVIN)

Riboflavin is necessary for red blood cell formation, antibody production, "cell respiration" and for growth in general. It alleviates all fatigue and is important in the prevention and treatment of cataracts. It aids in the metabolism of carbohydrates, fats and proteins. When used with Vitamin A, it maintains and improves the mucus membranes in the digestive tract. Riboflavin also facilitates oxygen use by the body tissues (skin and hair). Riboflavin can assist in eliminating dandruff and helps the uptake of Iron and Vitamin B_6 into the body. Vitamin B_2 is important during pregnancy because a lack of this vitamin may damage the fetus without the mother being aware of it. Vitamin B_2 is needed for the metabolism of tryptophan, which is converted to

Niacin in the body. Carpal tunnel syndrome or "Bible cyst" is improved from a program that includes Riboflavin and B6.

The reference to tryptophan needs comment here because tryptophan has been beaten up, knocked around and stomped on in recent years by the Food and Drug Administration (FDA). Tryptophan was implicated in some consumer toxic reaction deaths and pulled from the shelves. We have finally discovered that the FDA's indictment of tryptophan as being toxic in large doses was undeserved. Instead, the source of toxicity was due to the contaminants that were combined with tryptophan from a particular manufacturer.

Please note, however, that Caucasians who take large amounts of tryptophan as a sleep-inducer can experience a blood condition created by tryptophan known as "eosinophilia." Eosinophilia in Caucasians occurs because their brains (specifically, the pineal gland), which transform tryptophan into serotonin, leaves the blood stream with high amounts of serotonin. Why does this happen? Because Caucasians do not have enough melanocytes throughout their bodies to utilize the serotonin in the production of melanin. In the melanin-dominant races, tryptophan in unlimited amounts is immediately transformed and metabolized from serotonin to melanin. The serotonin is utilized by the brain to produce melanin-stimulating hormones. The more tryptophan melanin-dominant people eat, the more their brains (pituitary gland) can use it to produce stimulating hormones, thus enabling the melanocytes to produce melanin.

What about the eosinophilia disorder that occurs in Caucasians? Remember that I said that there are not enough melanocytes to relive the serotonin-saturated blood by converting the serotonin into melanin. In the formation of white blood cells, there is a particular white blood cells known as an eosinophil that carries serotonin within its cell structure. The eosinophil performs a very peculiar function in the body. It is used to stimulate increased blood circulation in an area of acute trauma. It also creates an immediate reaction in the body when foreign proteins or substances get into the body. It is responsible for the reactions that are seen in acute allergic responses. The reaction it creates is due to the little granules of serotonin that it carries. When serotonin comes in contact with tissues, it creates an irritating response (swelling, heat, itching, etc.) eosinophils will also increase their number when the body has a chronic infection due to the presence of parasites or a different type of external pathogen.

In Caucasians, after taking increased amounts of tryptophan, the serotonin circulating around in the blood must be removed or it will become toxic. The eosinophils will then absorb the serotonin and incorporate it into themselves. Now there is so much serotonin that the eosinophils must increase in number in an attempt to remove as much serotonin from the blood stream as possible to maintain balance or "homeostasis."

Now we have created a second problem. The first problem was the excess serotonin. The second problem is too many eosinophils. This causes a leukemic process because the presence of too many eosinophils decreases the amount of red blood cells that should be present in the circulatory system. Therefore, the necessary function that the red blood cells serve in the body is diminished in the face of the increased eosinophil population. This can be lethal, as physicians have seen in the past.

Now let us draw this part of the discussion to a focus. Given the above information, I feel the proper action by the FDA would have been to honor the ethnicity of race and to inform the public that Caucasians cannot tolerate tryptophan in high doses because of their melanocyte deficiency. Therefore,

Caucasians can safely take the proper amount of tryptophan and B vitamins without hurting themselves. However, the FDA need not deprive other ethnic or melanin-dominant races of what they need to sustain themselves. Melanin-dominant races require tryptophan to be healthy. They MUST have it!

I thought it was very interesting that, in admonishing the public about taking tryptophan, the FDA did not also inform them about the food sources that are high in tryptophan, such as spinach, carrots, and mushrooms. No recommendation was made to monitor or eliminate large quantities of these foods from the diet so as not to cause health problems for the Caucasian race.

Finally, back to Riboflavin It is indeed needed for the metabolism of tryptophan, which, as indicated earlier, is converted to Niacin in the body. This is only one pathway through which tryptophan is metabolized. Deficiency symptoms include cramps and sores at the corner of the mouth.

Sources

Vitamin B2 is found in beans, spinach, asparagus, avocados, Brussels sprouts, currents, nuts, and grains (e.g., wheat, wild rice).

Warning

Doctor recommendations that increase the need for riboflavin include oral contraceptives and strenuous exercise. Please note that the B vitamins in general can easily be destroyed by light, excess cooking, and alcohol ingestion.

It is also important to note that mounting research is indicating that Melanin Dominant people do not require this vitamin from external sources.

Some researchers are indicating that this vitamin is artificially produced from natural primary melanin pigments.

VITAMIN B3 (NIACIN, NIACINAMIDE)

Vitamin B3 is needed for proper circulation and healthy skin. Vitamin B3, commonly known as Niacin, aids in the function of the nervous system and the metabolism of carbohydrates, fats, proteins, and in the production of hydrochloric acid for the digestive system. Niacin lowers cholesterol and improves circulation. Niacin is also effective in the treatment of schizophrenia and other mental illnesses.

It is very interesting that this vitamin is not used at all or very little in institutions that house the psychologically imbalanced. If one reads these patients' hospital charts, one notices that very few are getting any vitamins at all, and many of them are using drugs such as nicotine in the form of cigarettes. Cigarette smoking definitely destroys B vitamins, especially Niacin, because of the heat and light sensitivity of this vitamin.

Sources

Niacin and niacinamide are found in broccoli, carrots, cauliflower, potatoes, tomatoes (but beware of eating potatoes and tomatoes, because they interfere with mid-brain activity), and whole wheat.

Let me comment a little more about potatoes and tomatoes. Both are in the "nightshade" family. They contain a common chemical known as "solanine." As members of the solanaceae species of plants, they are poisonous! "Cancer apple," was a common name for the tomato in many areas in Europe during the early 1900s. It was used only for ornamentation and seldom eaten because of its toxic effects. Potatoes were not eaten until after the rye famine and rye grain blight that occurred in Ireland in the 1700s. Because the rye plants were destroyed by blight, the tuberous potato plant was eaten as a temporary survival food. However, it remained and was brought to the United States during the migration period and has now become a mainstay in many households and in fast food restaurants across the country.

Be reminded that the potato and tomato interfere with mid-brain activity, and it is this very mid-brain function that is necessary for creative activity and conceptualization. Authors such as Rudolph Steiner have noted that the potato and tomato spiritually do not have much direction and that they tend to "amplify" the spiritual/mental characteristics of the foods with which they are combined. Thus, Steiner asserts in his writings that the potato and tomato augment the mental and spiritual vibrations of meat. This means that when these foods are eaten with meat, the impact on the body is like eating double portions of flesh!

Warning

Watch out for "flushing." Usually harmless, it occurs after the ingestion of Niacin. A red rash will appear on the skin and a tingling sensation may be experienced as well. How much Niacin should be used with caution by those who are pregnant, and those suffering from gout, peptic ulcer, glaucoma, liver disease and diabetes? When the lymphatic system is clean and open, you will not experience flushing. It has been my experience using clinical observation that flushing is a result of or indication of lymphatic and end capillary blockage. Drinking appropriate amounts of water, getting proper body massage, using a loofa sponge over the entire body, or dry skin brushing daily will stop the flushing and itching reactions when taking Niacin.

Etymologically, Nicotine is not a naturally occurring vitamin and is a breakdown product of Nicotine. Melanin dominant people do not require niacin as it has been identified to exist in classical nutrition.[1]

PANTOTHENIC ACID (B5)

Vitamin B5, called pantothenic acid, is also known as the anti-stress vitamin. It plays a role in the production of adrenaline, in reducing inflammations, and in the production of antibodies in the body. It also aids in vitamin utilization by the body. Pantothenic acid helps to convert fats, carbohydrates, and proteins into energy. This vitamin is noted to produce vital steroids and cortisone in the adrenal glands and is an essential component for enzyme activity. The body produces its own steroids via the adrenal glands.

Pantothenic acid is required by all cells of the body and is concentrated in the organs. It is needed for normal function of the digestive tract and may be helpful in treating depression and anxiety.

Sources

The following foods contain pantothenic acid: beans, mother's milk, fresh vegetables (almost all types), and whole wheat.

Warning

Most side effects have been documented. To date, I have not found any side effects, but will be alert to any possibilities.

---

[1] Research provided by Dr. LiNiViLi ZiMiLiZi, Brooklyn, New York, 1993

VITAMIN B6 (PYRIDOXINE)

Pyridoxine is involved in more bodily functions than any other nutrient. It affects both physical and mental health. It is beneficial if one suffers from water retention. This vitamin is necessary in the production of hydrochloric acid and the absorption of fats and proteins. For proper absorption of fats and proteins, one needs Vitamin B_6. Many persons have gall bladder and liver disease because they are pyridoxine deficient.

Pyridoxine assists in maintaining the sodium and potassium balance, and promotes red blood cell formation. For those who are hypertensive and are taking diuretics or hypertension medication, it is very important to make sure that there is sufficient pyridoxine supplementation in the diet. Many of these hypertension medications and diuretics cause an imbalance in both the sodium and potassium, which is why many persons are taking hypertension potassium supplements. Please check out your diet for pyridoxine; it could be seriously deficient.

Pyridoxine is also required by the nervous system and is needed for normal brain function and for the synthesis of RNA and DNA, that portion of cell structure that contains the genetic instructions for reproduction of all cells and for normal cellular function and growth.

It is extremely important that you understand that this vitamin is directly associated with the health of your genes. This genetic information that you carry within your body reflects seven generations of your mother's and father's sides of the family. This is a fantastic library that is walking around in your body, and you must keep it healthy. Pyridoxine is paramount to having healthy genes.

Call Vitamin B_6 the "Gene Vitamin." It activates many enzymes and aids in Vitamin B_{12}

absorption and antibody production. Vitamin B_6 has a role in cancer immunity and in arteriosclerosis. It inhibits the formation of a toxic chemical called homocysteine. This homocysteine attacks the heart muscle and allows the deposition of cholesterol in muscle to occur. B_6 is also useful in preventing kidney stones and acts as a mild diuretic.

Often in my clinical practice, I have seen hypertension patients who have little brown moles around the lower eyelids. What does that tell me? It tells me that they have kidney stones, most likely due to excessive pantothenic acid formation. It also tells me they are Vitamin B_6 deficient. Up to 90% of them are on anti-hypertension medication and are usually in some type of delicate potassium balance or imbalance.

So, now we know that B_6 also can prevent those kidney stones and that the lack of B_6 may be the reason why so many people have those moles on their faces. When B_6 is deficient, the individual does not produce enough hydrochloric acid and is not able to properly break down proteins. The proteins then get stuck in the lymphatic system and reappear on the surface of the skin as moles (technically called "seborrhea keratoses"). What these moles really show is protein and fat metabolic disease. Note: Vitamin B_6 reduces the symptoms of premenstrual syndrome and is helpful in treating allergies, arthritis and asthma.

Sources

All foods contain small amounts of Vitamin B_6. The following foods have the highest amounts: carrots, peas, spinach, sunflower seeds, walnuts, wheat germ, avocados, bananas, beans, blackstrap molasses (again), brown rice and other whole grains, cabbage and cantaloupe.

Warning

Antidepressives, estrogen, and oral contraceptives may increase the need for Vitamin B_6 in the body.

VITAMIN B_{12} (Cyanocobalamin)

Vitamin B_{12} (cyanocobalamin) is needed to prevent anemia (a special kind called "pernicious anemia") Vitamin B_{12} aids in cellular longevity. This vitamin is required for proper digestion, absorption of food, protein synthesis, and metabolism of carbohydrates and fats. In addition, Vitamin B_{12} prevents nerve damage, maintains virility, and promotes normal growth and development.

Vitamin B_{12} deficiencies can be caused by malabsorption due to improper hydrochloric acid production in the stomach lining, and also due to a deficiency of a substance known as "intrinsic factor." Deficient intrinsic factor is a very common problem in the elderly and in those with digestive disorders.

Vegetarians are also more likely to have this deficiency if they do not eat fermented foods. Yet, it can be reliably said that vegetarian eating is the normal mode of nourishment for the largest population of the human race on this planet. The melanin-dominant race is, in fact, the largest population of people on the planet, and they are, by genetic heritage, vegetarians. Being a vegetarian requires that one has the appropriate flora in the digestive tract. Why? Because these bacteria live in a symbiotic relationship with us. B_{12} is produced in small amounts by the bacteria in our intestine. We then absorb B_{12}, which is utilized as needed in metabolic reactions or else stored by our liver. This is why fermented foods in the diet of melanin-dominant individuals are so important. Fermented foods include pickles (long and short-term), as well as fermented beets in the form of tempeh or natto.

Deficiency symptoms of B_{12} include abnormal gout, memory loss, hallucinations, eye disorders, anemia, and digestive disorders.

Sources

The largest amounts of Vitamin B_{12} are found in fermented foods such as fermented vegetables, picked foods such as cucumbers, tempeh, natto, and miso. Other sources of B_{12} located in animal products and cheeses that are more appropriate sources of B_{12} for the Caucasian race.

Warning

Anti-gout medication, anticoagulant drugs, and potassium supplements may block absorption of B12 in the digestive tract.

BIOTIN

Biotin aids in cell growth, fatty acid production, and the metabolism of carbohydrates and proteins, and any utilization of the B-complex vitamins.

Sufficient quantities are needed for healthy hair and skin. This is why we see biotin shampoos and biotin added into nail care cosmetics. Biotin may prevent hair loss in some individuals. Biotin also promotes healthy sweat glands, muscle tissue and bone marrow.

I would like to comment on bone marrow here. Please understand that healthy red blood cells are not made from the bone marrow. They are made directly from the villus of the small intestines, DIRECTLY FROM THE FOOD THAT WE EAT! Only in disease does the bone marrow contribute any significant amounts of red blood cells or blood to the circulatory system. This is such a broad subject that ten volumes of research have been done in Japan over the last 30 years. Yet, to this day, none of it has been honored by physicians, hematologists and most health commissions in the Western medical field. The link to the digestive tract has been grossly overlooked. Know that healthy blood is determined by the health of the digestive tract.

Now back to biotin. The deficiency of the B vitamin is rare because it can be produced in the intestine from fruit. However, the modern overuse of synthetic foods - the type that has no life force energy - has negatively affected biotin synthesis. The bacteria of the intestines do not attempt to metabolize synthetic food. As a result, biotin production is becoming a problem for some. Those individuals who continue to eat living foods (as opposed to canned, frozen, packaged or freeze dried) will not be biotin-deficient. The major bacterium known to man that should be in the intestinal tract is known as "Acidophilus Buffans." This bacterium has been found to give us the highest amount of biotin and B_{12} for absorption by our intestines.

Sources of biotin are acidophilus, as mentioned, which may be taken in the form of non-dairy soybean (especially soybean tempeh), whole grains, and yeast.

Warning

Raw egg whites contain a protein called "avidin," which combines with biotin in the intestinal tract and depletes the body of biotin. By now you know that melanin-dominant individuals should not eat raw eggs. Women, especially, are cautioned against eating raw eggs.

In the Caucasian race eating raw eggs is quite common and it appears that Caucasians are able to endure biotin deficiencies. This protein overdose combines with B_{12} and makes it unabsorbable. A dry, scaly scalp and/or face in infants (seborrheic dermatitis) may indicate a deficiency. Look at the cheeks of your children. If they look dry, scaly, etc., suspect biotin deficiency.

We see this quite commonly in Caucasian children who have very dry, scaly pink cheeks. Consuming rancid fat inhibits biotin absorption.

For those who are still eating "Sweet and Low," which is saccharin, you know right now you have a problem. I would not be surprised that this is also a problem with aspartame or "NutraSweet." Do not eat products that contain artificial sweeteners or salt substitutes. We are now discovering that these ingredients cause havoc in the body. If you must have sugar, use maple syrup, rice honey or barley malt. Even white sugar is more appropriate than any of the synthetic sweeteners. Clear your body of the harassment and disorder that these things create. Remember the cyclamates? They, too, were thought to be just wonderful. Twenty years later we found that they were causing all kinds of cancers and problems. This is going to be the same problem with using aspartame or NutraSweet. Stay away from these additives, and please read the labels because they are contained in many foods.

Finally, note that the use of sulfur drugs or antibiotics threatens the availability of biotin for use in the body.

CHOLINE

Choline is needed for 1) nerve transmission, 2) gall bladder regulation, 3) liver function, and 4) lecithin formation. It minimizes excess fat in the liver, aids in hormone production, and is necessary in fat and cholesterol metabolism. Without choline, brain function and memory are impaired.

Choline is beneficial for disorders of the nervous system such as Parkinson's disease and tardive dyskinesia. Tardive dyskinesia is a peculiarity of behavior brought on by the prolonged use of psychotropic medication. The symptoms are seen in people who walk around the streets constantly sticking their tongues out, or constantly blinking their eyes. Their fingers move as if they were mimicking a little bird chirping, or as if they were playing castanets. We, as clinicians, often see this in individuals who are taking phenothiazine drugs. These drugs are commonly known as Thorazine, Haldol, and Prolixin, drugs typically prescribed for schizophrenics and manic depressives in our psychiatric institutions. Prolonged use produces the side-effect of tardive dyskinesia, a condition due to phenothiazine toxicity. Another drug, Cogentin, is usually given to help balance the side-effects of the phenothiazine toxicity.

It is interesting to note that tardive dyskinesia is not caused by phenothiazine toxicity alone. It may also be caused by choline deficiency that results in the build-up of fat in the liver. We are noticing that the institutions that house our psychologically impaired individuals are not giving them choline as a dietary supplement while the patients are taking these drugs on a daily basis. The question is, Why?

Sources

The sources for choline are beans and whole grain cereals. Why are the institutions that house our psychologically impaired not feeding the patients meals that consist primarily of whole grains and beans? Have you seen the menus lately? They consist of foods that come out of a can, that are frozen, and that often are years old. Interestingly, many of the patients never get better.

Warning

Eating a diet that is low in whole grains and beans can produce this deficiency. As stated, the ingestion of phenothiazine drugs for long periods of time can produce this deficiency, which may also, secondarily, reinforce tardive dyskinesia activity.

FOLIC ACID

Considered a brain food, folic acid is needed for energy production and formation of red blood cells. Folic Acid is a co-enzyme in DNA synthesis. It is important for healthy cell division and replication. It is involved in protein metabolism and has been used in the prevention and treatment of folic Acid anemia.

This nutrient may also help depression and anxiety and may be effective in the treatment of uterine cervical dysplasia. So, for those ladies who have had abnormal Pap smears, Class II or Class III cervical dysplasia, the treatment for the cervix is often laser therapy (or a more obsolete procedure called conization). Yet, therapists may not have increased the folic acid intake or asked the patient to eat foods high in folic acid. Perhaps these therapists need to be asked if they really understand all that is necessary for the physical body to heal itself with this condition.

Whatever the case, remember that if you are experiencing abnormal Pap indicating a possibility of developing uterine cancer, then folic acid is your best friend.

Folic acid also helps regulate the development of embryonic and fetal nerve cells. It is vital for normal growth and development of the fetus. Folic acid does best when combined with Vitamin B_{12}. A sore, red tongue is one sign of this deficiency. If you have eaten foods that are too acid-producing and so irritating to your tongue that it becomes sore and red, your folic acid is probably low.

Sources

Significant quantities of folic acid can be found in barley, beans, bran, brewer's yeast, whole grains (especially brown rice), dark green leafy vegetables, oranges, split peas, all root vegetables, carrots, parsnips, turnips, wheat germ, and yeast. People often purchase folic acid at the pharmacy, not realizing it is readily available dark green leafy vegetables. Please note that we do not eat raw salads and many raw vegetables in the winter time in the temperate zone. These foods contain too much water, tend to lower the body temperature, and can injure the kidneys. Be aware that raw foods are for spring, summer, and early fall never winter in the temperate zone.

Warning

Oral contraceptives may increase the need for folic acid. High doses used for extended periods should be avoided with a hormone related cancer or convulsive disorder. Why? Because folic acid can inhibit some of the hormones that have been used to treat certain cancers, and certain drugs, such as Dilantin, that are used to control seizure disorders, are neutralized by folic acid.

INOSITOL

Inositol is vital for hair growth. It helps prevent hardening of the arteries and is important in lecithin formation as well as fat and cholesterol metabolism. It helps remove fat from the liver.

Sources

Inositol is found in fruits, vegetables, and whole grains. Milk and meat sources also contain inositol. Remember milk and meat sources are not appropriate for melanin-dominant race.

Warning

Drinking large amounts of caffeine may cause a shortage of inositol in the body.

PARA-AMINOBENZOIC ACID (PABA)

Para-aminobenzoic acid, known as PABA, is one of the basic constituents of folic acid and helps with the utilization of pantothenic acid. This antioxidant helps protect against sunburn and skin cancers, and acts as co-enzymes. Co-enzymes help in the breakdown of protein and assist in the formation of red blood cells. Supplementing the diet with PABA may restore gray hair to its original color if the gray was created by stress or nutritional deficiencies. PABA content is very high in many of the sea vegetables. This is why sea vegetables, along with their high mineral content, have the capacity to restore the natural color to hair.

Sources

Molasses and whole grains are good sources for PABA.

Warning

Sulfur drugs may cause a deficiency of PABA.

BIOFLAVONOIDS

Some authors feel that bioflavonoids are not true vitamins in the strictest sense. However, we refer to them as a part of the B vitamins, and they are also known as Vitamin P. Bioflavonoids enhance the absorption of Vitamin C, and they should be taken together. They are always present in natural food sources high in Vitamin C. There are many products that list various bioflavonoids, including hesperetin, hesperidin, eriodictyon, quercetin and rutin. Whether the human body can produce bioflavonoids is a moot subject. They are used extensively in athletic injuries because they relieve pain of bumps and bruises. They also reduce pain located in the leg or across the back unless the symptoms are associated with prolonged bleeding and low serum calcium. Bioflavonoids act synergistically with Vitamin C to protect and preserve the structure of capillary blood vessels. In addition, bioflavonoids have an antibacterial effect and promote circulation, stimulate bowel production, lower cholesterol level, and treat and prevent cataracts. When taking Vitamin C, bioflavonoids also reduce the symptoms of oral herpes. Quercetin, found in algae, is a supplement that effectively treats asthma. Bromelin and querticin are synergistic and should be taken together to enhance absorption. Take 1000 mg of querticin daily and 3-6 doses for asthma or allergies. I have found a wonderful source of bioflavonoids in the form of concentrated rose hips and as a produce Bioflavonoid syrup. This helps with hemorrhoids and relieves thrombophlebitis, which is blood clots in the veins. It also helps to alleviate the condition of varicose veins.

Sources

The white material just beneath the peel of citrus fruits, peppers (especially red peppers), buckwheat and black currants contain bioflavonoids. Sources of Vitamin P include apricots, grapefruit, cherries, grapes, lemons, oranges, prunes and rose hips.

Warning

Extremely high doses may cause diarrhea.

Nutrients & Dosages

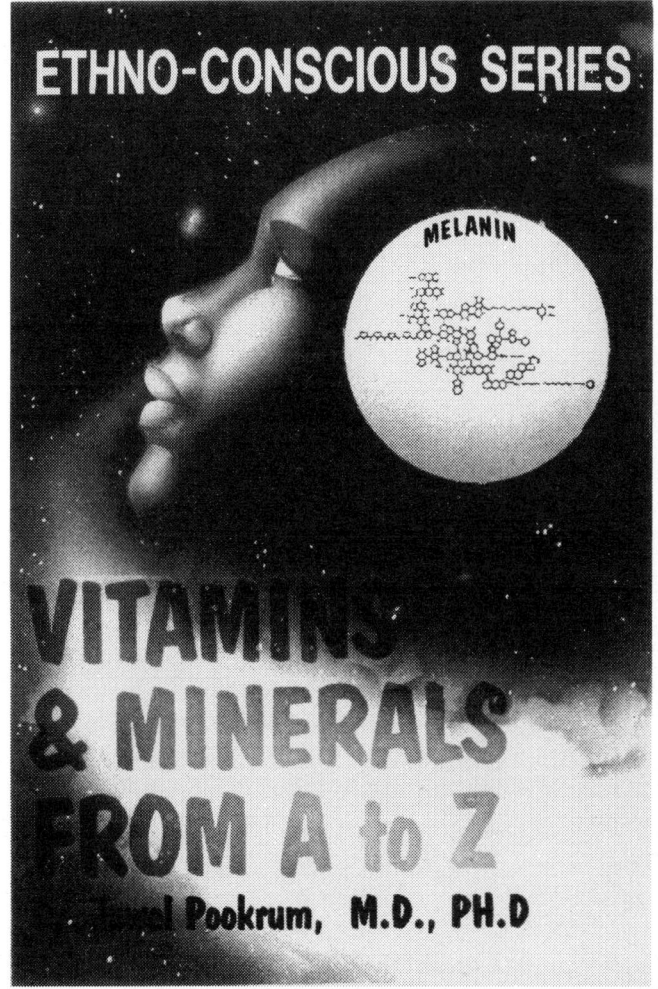

For Good health

NUTRIENTS & DOSAGES FOR MAINTAINING GOOD HEALTH

The nutrients listed below are recommended for good health. Daily dosages are suggested; however, before using any supplements, you should consult your physician. Dosages will vary according to age, weight, and ethnicity.

Note: The following list has been established for the Caucasian race. Updates for melanin-dominant race are being compiled. For specific dosages, please contact your nutritionist or physician of nutritional medicine.

Vitamins	Daily Dosages
Beta-Carotene	15,000 IU
Vitamin A	10,000 IU
Vitamin D	400 IU
Vitamin E	600 IU
Vitamin K (alfalfa)	100 mcg
Vitamin C (with the mineral ascorbates)	3,000 mg
Bioflavonoids	500 mg
Hesperidin	100 mg
Rutin	25 mg

Vitamins	Daily Dosages
Folic Acid	400 mcg
Thiamine (B1)	50 mg
Riboflavin (B2)	50 mg
Niacin	100 mg
Niacinamide	100 mg
Vitamin B_6 (pyridoxine)	50 mg
Vitamin B_{12} (cyanocobalamin)	300 mcg
Biotin	300 mcg
Choline	100 mg
Inositol	100 mg
Para-Aminobenzoic Acid (PABA)	25 mg
Vitamin F (unsaturated fatty acids)	

Minerals	Daily Dosages
Calcium (chelate)	1,500 mg
Chromium (GTF)	150 mcg
Copper	3 mg
Iodine (kelp)	225 mcg
Iron*	18 mg
Magnesium	750 mg
Manganese	2 mg
Molybdenum	30 mcg
Potassium	99 mg
Selenium	200 mcg
Zinc	30 mg

Optional Supplements	Daily Dosages
Co-enzyme Q$_{10}$	30 mg
Garlic (Kyolic)	
Germanium Ge-32	60 mg
L-Carnitine	100 mg
L-Cysteine	50 mg
L-Lysine	50 mg
L-Methionine	50 mg
L-Tyrosine	100 mg
Lecithin	200 - 500 mg
Pectin	50 mg
RNA-DNA	50 mg
Silicon	
Superoxide dismutase (SOD)	

* Iron should be taken separately, but may be omitted if no deficiency exists. Do not take Iron in multisupplement formula.

Minerals

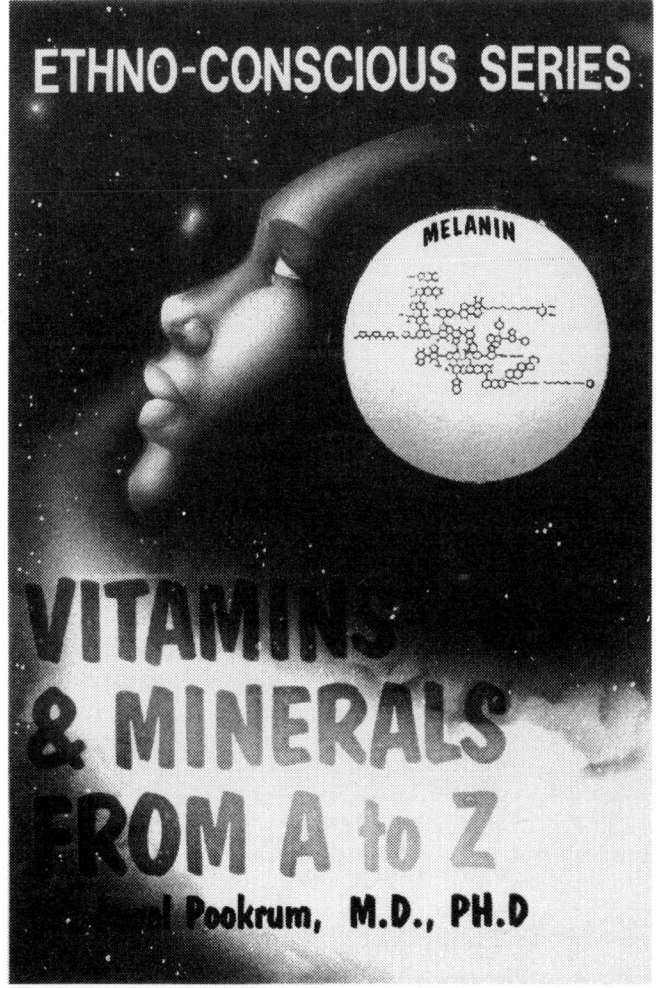

MINERALS

THE FUNCTION OF MINERALS

Minerals function as coenzymes, enabling the body to quickly and accurately perform its activities. They are needed for the proper composition of body fluids, formation of blood and bones, and the maintenance of healthy nerve function. Minerals are naturally occurring elements found in the earth. The earth is the foundation for all life forms on the planet; therefore, all plants and animals also contain minerals. Minerals form the foundation of the skeletal system within the body of the organism whether plant or animal.

Rocks are made up of mineral salts. As rocks and stones are broken down into tiny fragments by years of erosion, dust and sand accumulate, forming the basis of soil. Beside these tiny crystals of mineral salts, the soil is teeming with microorganisms that utilize them. The minerals are then passed from the soil to the plants, which in turn are eaten by herbivorous animals. Man ingests these minerals when he consumes plants or plant-eating animals.

Minerals belong to two groups: macrominerals or bulk minerals, and microminerals or trace minerals. Bulk minerals include calcium, magnesium, sodium, potassium, and phosphorus. These are needed in larger amounts than are the trace minerals. Although only minute amounts of trace minerals are needed, they are important for good health. Trace minerals include zinc, Iron, copper, manganese, chromium, selenium and iodine. Because minerals are stored primarily in the body's bones and muscle tissue, it is possible to overdose on minerals if an extremely large does is taken. Toxic amounts accumulate only if massive amounts are taken for a prolonged of time.

IMPROVING MINERAL ABSORPTION

Most minerals are normally obtained through the foods that we eat. As we stated earlier, the plants that are eaten have minerals in their cellular system, and as we eat these plants, small amounts of minerals are absorbed into our bodies. Minerals are not free floating in either plants or animals; they are normally attached to something, usually a protein. This attachment is called chelation. We have found that minerals are absorbed much better when they are attached to a protein and can enter more easily into the blood stream. When minerals are not chelated (attached to a protein), they can accumulate in various body tissues or clog up certain body organs and create problems. Normally, when minerals are not chelated in the healthy body, they are eliminated through the urine. If one has become mineral deficient, mineral supplements should be taken with meals that contain protein to allow chelation of the mineral for easier absorption. When taking mineral supplements, use the chelated form.

Orotated minerals also work quite well in that the asporotate addition to the mineral allows it be absorbed with ease. Minerals are chelated when they are combined with orotic acids. The charge that is attached to the mineral when it becomes chelated with orotic acids causes the outer cell membranes to readily absorb the mineral. The Food and Drug Administration has called for the removal of orotated minerals from the market. This decision is particularly disheartening because my experience is that they work quite well, even better than the chelated protein form of minerals. It is still not clear why the FDS has requested the removal of the orotated minerals.

Once a mineral is absorbed, it must get from the blood into the cells, and then be transferred across the cell membranes in a form that can be utilized by the cell. After the minerals enter the body, they compete with other minerals for absorption; therefore minerals should always be taken in balanced amounts. For example, too much zinc can deplete the body of copper, and excessive calcium intake can affect magnesium absorption. In addition, fiber decreases the body's absorption of minerals; therefore, take supplemental fiber and minerals at different times. If taken together, the fiber will absorb the minerals, hold it within itself, and pass through the body without being absorbed.

CALCIUM

Calcium is vital in the formation of strong bones and teeth, and it is important in the maintenance of regular heartbeat and the transmission of nerve impulses. It is needed for muscle growth and contraction and the prevention of muscle cramp. This important mineral is also essential in blood clotting and helps prevent cancer of the colon. It can lower blood pressure and prevent bone loss, especially osteoporosis. Calcium provides energy and participates in the protein structure of RNA and DNA. It also improves the activation of several enzymes including lactase, which is necessary for the absorption of fat. The amino acid lysine is needed for calcium absorption.

Calcium protects bones and teeth from lead by inhibiting this toxic metal. If there is a calcium deficiency, lead will be absorbed by the body and deposited in the teeth and bones. This may account for the higher levels of lead in children who have a higher incidence of cavities. A calcium deficiency may result in the following symptoms: muscle cramps. nervousness, heart palpitations, brittle nails, eczema, hypertension, aching joints, increased cholesterol levels, rheumatoid arthritis, tooth decay, insomnia, rickets and numbness in the arm and leg.

Calcium is more effective when taken in smaller doses spread throughout the day and before bedtime. Always note that calcium should be taken in its natural sources. For melanin-dominant individuals, it is always through eating an abundance of dark green leafy vegetables that are not overcooked. When taken at night, calcium tends to produce a sound sleep. Female athletes and women experiencing menopause need greater amounts of calcium due to lower estrogen level. Estrogen protects the skeletal system by promoting the deposit of calcium into the bones.

Sources

Calcium is found in green leafy vegetables, almonds, asparagus, blackstrap molasses, brewer's yeast, broccoli, cabbage, carob, collard greens, dandelion greens, filberts, dulse, kale, kelp, mustard greens, oats, parsley, seeds, tofu, turnip greens, prunes and hijiki. Hijiki sea vegetables are the highest source of calcium known to man. A 2-ounce serving contains 1,000 ml of calcium; an 8-ounce glass of milk contains only 300 ml, mucus and possible diseases.

Oxalic acid found in soy beans, kale, rhubarb, greens, almonds, cashews, chard, cocoa and especially spinach, interferes with calcium absorption by binding with calcium in the intestines and producing insoluble salts that cannot be absorbed. Casual consumption of foods with oxalic acid should not pose a problem; however, over indulging prohibits the absorption of calcium. What does this mean? Melanin-dominant individuals should eat foods such as sea vegetables alone, not mixed with other foods. This eliminates the oxalic acid competition. Is it not interesting that people who eat chocolates obviously will become calcium deficient? Please note that almonds have only a minimum amount of oxalic acid, while spinach is extremely high in oxalic acid. For this reason we do not recommend the consumption of spinach on a frequent basis.

Calcium supplements should not be taken by those with kidney stones or kidney disease. Calcium may interfere with the effects of verapamil, a channel blocker of the heart. Tums as a source of calcium neutralizes the stomach acid needed for calcium absorption; however, we realize this is a very abnormal source of calcium, even though it has been recommended by many physicians. I feel that Tums is a very inferior calcium source when a proper diet is not recommended in conjunction. Calcium taken with Iron reduces the effect of both minerals, and too much calcium can interfere with the absorption of zinc, just as zinc can interfere with calcium absorption. A hair analysis can determine the levels of these two minerals in your body if you have questions regarding calcium/zinc levels.

Insufficient Vitamin D intake or excessive phosphorus and magnesium can hinder the intake of calcium. Although heavy exercise also hinders calcium uptake, moderate exercising contributes to its uptake. The diet that is high either in protein, fat or sugar also negatively affects calcium uptake and had been found to be the cause of osteoporosis. If you eat too much protein, brittle, spongy bones will result. So many women in our society are taking calcium pills because they are afraid of osteoporosis.

What they need to do is stop eating flesh, especially if they are of a melanin-dominant race. The female species of that race is never to indulge in meat eating. They average American diet, composed of meat, refined grains, and soft drinks high in phosphorus, leads to increased bone loss and decreased growth. Foods such as vegetables, fruits and whole grains, which contain significant amounts of calcium but lower amounts of phosphorus, should be consumed.

IRON

Perhaps the most important function of Iron is its production of hemoglobin and oxygenation of red blood cells. Iron is the mineral found in the largest amounts in the blood. This mineral is essential for many enzymes, and is important for growth in children and resistance to disease. Iron is also required for a healthy immune system and for energy production. Vitamin C can increase our absorption as much as 30%. Iron deficiency symptoms include brittle hair, nails that are spoonshaped or that have ridges running lengthwise, hair loss, fatigue, paleness, dizziness and anemia.

Sufficient hydrochloric acid production must be present in the stomach in order for iron to be absorbed. Copper, manganese, molybdenum, Vitamin A and B-complex vitamins are also needed for complete iron absorption. General medical books state that iron utilization is impaired by rheumatoid arthritis and cancer in the liver. iron deficiency anemia occurs despite ample amounts of iron stored in the liver, spleen and bone marrow. Recent medical journals also state that Iron deficiency is prevalent in those suffering from candidiasis, which is a chronic fungal infection, and chronic herpes infection.

Excess Iron buildup in the tissues has been associated with the rare disease known as hemochromatosis, a disease characterized by bronze skin pigmentation, sclerosis, diabetes, and heart disorders. It is noted that hemochromatosis is not common in melanin-dominant race.

Sources

Iron is found in green leafy vegetables, whole grains, enriched whole grain breads, and cereals.

Other food sources include avocados, beets, blackstrap molasses, brewer's yeast, dulse, kelp, kidney and lima beans, millet, parsley, peaches, pears, dried prunes, pumpkins, raisins, rice and wheat bran, sesame seeds, and soybeans.

Warning

Excess amounts of zinc and Vitamin E interfere with Iron absorption. Those who engage in strenuous exercise and who perspire heavily deplete iron stored in the body. Excess iron stored in the body can cause problems. Increased iron in the tissues can lead to the production of free radicals and an increased need for Vitamin E.

Iron deficiency may result from intestinal bleeding, from excessive menstrual bleeding, a diet high in phosphorus (such as soda pop), poor digestion, long-term illness, ulcers, prolonged use of antacids, excess coffee, or tea containing caffeine. See your medical doctor to investigate these symptoms before prescribing iron for yourself. In some cases doctors have discovered that an anemia is not always due to iron deficiency, but can be due to B_6 or B_{12} deficiencies. According to a 1988 medical journal, one should not take extra iron if one has an infection because bacteria require iron to grow. The body stores iron and does not utilize it when there is an infection. Taking extra iron merely feeds the bacteria.

ZINC

This essential mineral is important in prostate gland function and in the growth of the reproductive organs. It is required for protein synthesis and collagen formation, and promotes a healthy immune system necessary for the healing of wounds. Zinc also allows acuity of taste and smell and protects the liver from chemical damage. It is interesting that we find that the loss of smell and taste occurs most commonly in men. Urinary complaints and prostate disease are usually due to a zinc deficiency that has not been recognized by the treating physician or nutritionist. Sufficient intake and absorption of zinc is needed in order to maintain the proper concentration of Vitamin E in the blood.

Sources

Zinc is found in the following foods: legumes, seas food, seaweeds, nuts, and whole grains. Significant quantities of zinc are also found in brewer's yeast, lima beans, liver, mushrooms, pecans, pumpkin seeds, soy lecithin, soy beans, sunflower seeds and tourla.

Warning

Dosages of more than 100 mg of zinc can depress the immune system; doses of 100 mg and under can enhance the immune response. Zinc levels may be lowered by diarrhea, kidney disease, cirrhosis of the liver, diabetes and ingestion of extra fiber. The phytates found in grains and some beans bind with zinc so that it cannot be absorbed. The proper copper and zinc balance should be maintained. Consumption of hard water can upset the zinc levels.

COPPER

Copper was recognized around 1875 as a normal constituent of human blood. It is in highest concentrations in liver, brain, heart, and kidney tissue. It has been noted that muscle tissue has the lowest concentration, but due to the muscle percentage of the total body, muscle contains over 40% of the entire concentration of copper in the body.

Function

Copper is a component of the major enzymes of the body. When there is copper deficiency, there is almost total enzyme failure. Copper has a very important role in the oxidation of the Iron before its transport in the plasma and in the collagen binding process to aid wound healing. It plays an important role in energy production in all the cells in the body, assists in the protection of the body from antioxidants, and, most of all, is strategic in the production of melanin and adrenal hormones.

Transport

Copper is absorbed from the stomach, but in maximal amounts through the small intestines. It is noted that the more copper one eats, the less is absorbed. Copper is carried through the body attached to a few forms of protein. It is stored within the liver and is excreted from the liver in bile. Copper is lost from the body in sweat, urine and menstrual blood.

Peculiarity

Copper is one of those strange elements of which a little goes a long way. The more copper you take, the less you absorb. It is also important that when eating foods with high concentrations of copper, large quantities of other minerals are not present. For example, taking too much zinc will create a copper deficiency. Men attempting to increase their virility by taking large amounts of zinc may create a copper deficiency, thus creating a health problem. The recommended daily amount is 2 mg/day of zinc. Taking 150 mg/day can be excessive and create a significant copper deficiency.

Additionally, copper is a very important trace mineral for the melanin-dominant race. Without this, melanin production is almost impossible. Copper must be present in adequate amounts in the body for adequate iron absorption.

Anemia, low white blood cell counts, bone hemorrhages, hair and skin depigmentation (loss of color), wrinkled skin, and brain degeneration are all due in large part to copper deficiencies. When children have low white blood cell counts, think first of copper deficiency, not leukemia. It is also possible that many cases of vitiligo are due to copper deficiencies.

Sources

Nuts, dried beans, whole cereal grains, dried fruits, and shellfish are major sources of copper. It has been noted that cow's milk is a very poor source of copper. Human mother's milk is a much better and healthier source of copper for infants because it is very well absorbed.

SELENIUM

Selenium is a vital antioxidant, especially when combined with Vitamin E. As an antioxidant, selenium protects the immune system by preventing the formation of free radicals, which can damage the body. Selenium and Vitamin E act synergistically to aid in production of antibodies and to help maintain a healthy heart. This trace element is needed for pancreatic function and tissue elasticity. A selenium deficiency has been linked to cancer and heart disease.

In New Zealand, soils are low in selenium. The cattle and sheep there experience breakdowns in muscle tissue, including the heart muscle. However, human intake of selenium there is adequate because of Australian wheat imports. For those individuals, especially Caucasians who eat beef and lamb imported from New Zealand and who rely upon this flesh to provide selenium, there is the danger they could become selenium deficient. However, because of the wheat import, they are able to overcome local selenium deficiency.

Sources

Depending on the soil content, selenium can be found in wheat and grain. It can also be found in Brazil nuts, brewer's yeast, broccoli, chicken, dairy products, garlic, liver, molasses, onions salmon and other seafoods, tourla, vegetables, wheat germ and whole grains.

Warning

No dangers have been noted to date.

ALUMINUM

Aluminum has been found to be toxic. It permeates our air, water and soil, and small amounts are present in our foods. The average person consumes between 3 and 10 mg of aluminum per day. Only recently have researchers learned that aluminum is absorbed and accumulated in the body. Aluminum is a popular metal used to make cookware, cooking utensils, and foil. Excessive use of antacids is the most common source of aluminum in the body. Mylanta, Maalox, Gelusil, Amphojel and many others have a high aluminum content. Many of the over the counter drugs used for inflammation and pain contain aluminum, including Anacin arthritis pain formula, Ascriptin, Bufferin, and Vanquish. Douche preparations such as Massengill and Summer Eve contain aluminum.

Let me just comment on Massengill. Having been trained as a gynecologist, I could always tell by looking at a woman's vagina if she used Massengill because it always left tiny bumps on the surface, as if somebody stamped a little suction pad over the mucous and left little lumps throughout the vagina. There was no accompanying pain or excess discharge, but I feel it is not healthy, in the long term, to continue to use a douche preparation that would alter the contour of the mucus membrane to the point it took on a granular patterning. Could it have been aluminum?

Aluminum is also an additive in most baking powders and is sometimes evident in drinking water. We recommend that you use Rumford baking powder. This is the only baking powder of which we are aware that does not contain aluminum and still has the double acting rising potential.

Many symptoms of aluminum toxicity are similar to Alzheimer's disease and osteoporosis. Aluminum toxicity can lead to colic, rickets, gastric-

liver and kidney function, forgetfulness, speech disturbances, memory loss, and softening of the bones. Weak, aching muscles can also be present. Research suggests that chronic calcium deficiency may change the way in which the body uses minerals, including aluminum. Bone loss and increased intestinal absorption of aluminum and silicon combine to form compounds that accumulate in the cerebral cortex of the brain. These compounds prevent impulses from being carried to and from the brain.

An accumulation of aluminum salts in the brain has been implicated in seizures and reduced mental faculties. Autopsies performed on Alzheimer's victims reveal that four times the normal amount of aluminum had accumulated in the nerve cells in the brain. This reflects that bone accumulation of aluminum in the brain may contribute to the development of Alzheimer disease.

The Caucasian race, which generally prefers the taste of meat, should be aware that aluminum is added to processed cheese for its melting qualities for use on hamburgers.

GOLD

This is the emperor of all metals. It is a beautiful metal to the eye, but also has tremendous effects on the body. Modern medicine has discovered that gold has the capacity to regenerate tissue, especially joint tissue, and has been using gold for many years as a therapy for arthritis. However, the amount of gold used was quite high relative to the real needs of the body, and in many instances created toxicity. When gold is taken at very, very dilute levels, as in homeopathic therapy, it regenerates all tissues and energizes the life force. This is especially true in the melanin-dominant race.

Gold has also been used and found to be destructive to cancer cells; it has been used with and as a form of chemotherapeutic agent. Again the concentration has been rather high, and has been known to be toxic. Because gold is so inert, it is not absorbed very well by the body and it appears best results are obtained when used homeopathically or in minute amounts absorbed through the skin.

Halogens

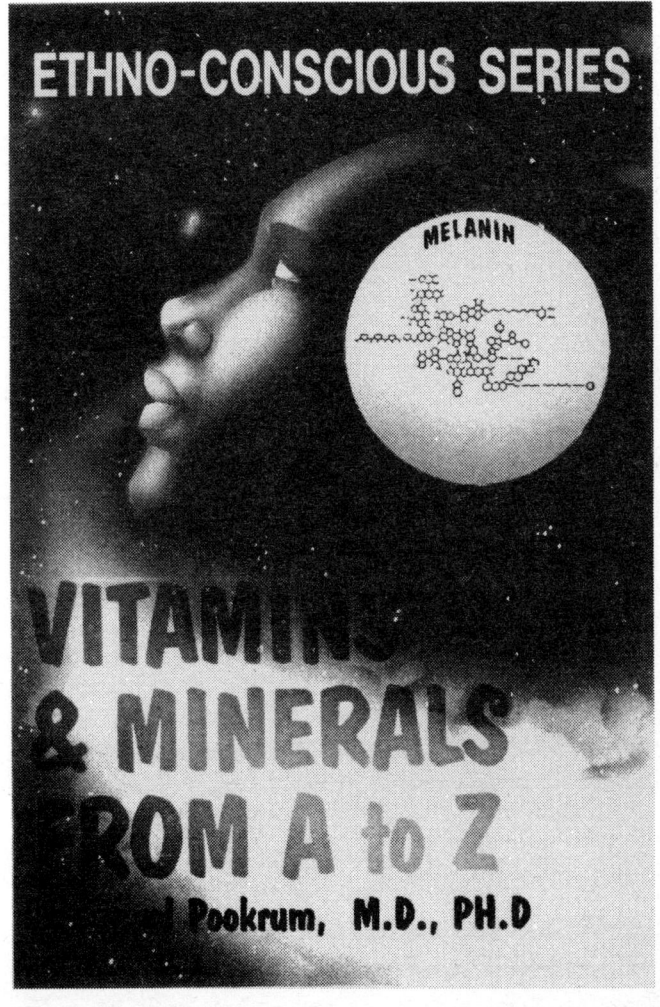

HALOGENS

FLUORINE

Fluorine belongs to the family of elements known as halogens. When we think of fluorine, we normally think of water. For years controversy has raged over whether fluorides should be added to drinking water. Opponents say that fluorides occur naturally and help develop and maintain strong bones and teeth. Opponents to fluoridation contend that toxic levels of fluorine, the poisonous substance in fluorides, is derived from buildup in the body and causes irreparable harm to the immune system. Today, more than half of the cities in the United States add fluorine to their water supply. Although many ailments and disorders have been linked to fluoridated water (such as Downs Syndrome, molded teeth and cancer), fluoridation has become the standard rather than the exception. Should your tap water contain fluorine and you wish to remove it, a reverse osmosis or distillation system will eliminate almost all of the fluoride from the water. I recommend you use a clean water source without fluorine. Fluorine is needed in very, very small trace amounts to temper bones and to keep them from becoming brittle. The amount in many water systems is quite toxic and is causing many problems.

IODINE

Iodine is needed in only trace amounts. Iodine helps to metabolize excess fat and is important in physical and mental development. Iodine is needed for healthy thyroid glands and in the prevention of goiter. Mental retardation may result from an iodine deficiency in children. An iodine deficiency has been linked to BREAST CANCER. So it is very important for all breast cancer patients to take kelp or proper iodine supplements.

Sources

Foods high in iodine include sea vegetables such as hijiki, arame, dulse, kombu (kelp), and mekabu. It may also be found in asparagus, garlic, mushrooms, soy beans, summer squash and turnip greens.

Warning

Some foods block the uptake of iodine into the thyroid glands when eaten raw in large amounts. These include Brussels sprouts, cabbage, cauliflower, peaches, pears, spinach and turnips. If a hypothyroid disorder is present, eliminate the above vegetables from your diet. Excess iodine, over 30 times the recommended adult allowance, produces a metallic taste and sores in the mouth, swollen salivary glands, diarrhea and vomiting

Summary & References

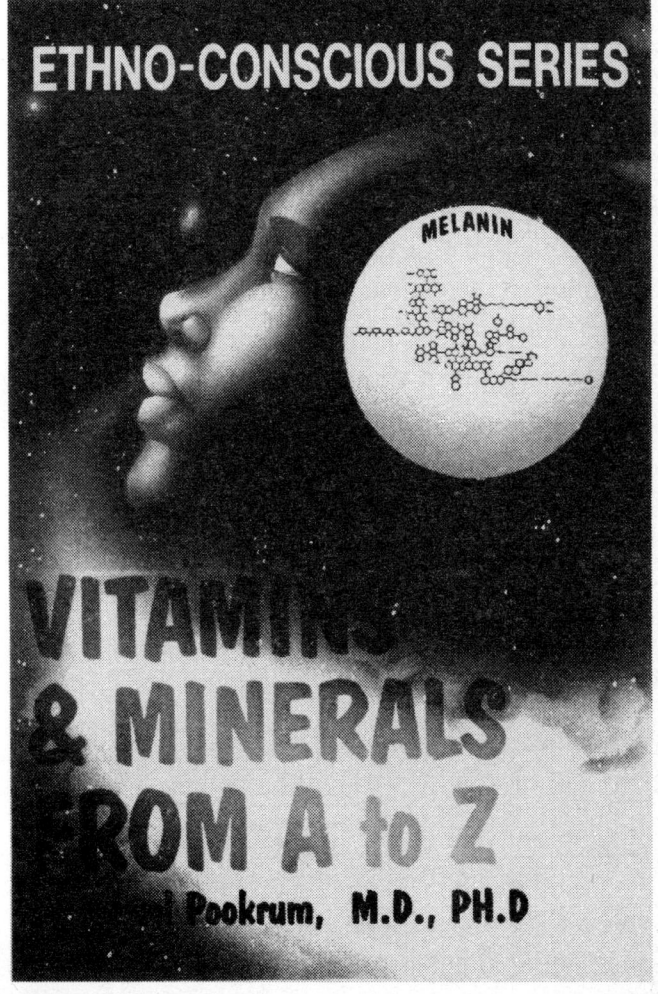

SUMMARY

It is noted that minerals and vitamins and how they are used is dependent upon individual needs, the requirements of the environment that one lives in, and an individual's daily activity. It is also important to note that ethnicity determines what minerals and vitamins should or should not be used. The duration of use and quantities are determined ethnically. Regardless of what race you are, it is important for you to study yourself, to understand how you relate to the external environment and to the change in the day, week, month and yearly cycles. You must understand that whether you are female or male determines the requirements of your body, and any program of nutritional supplementation must take this into account.

If you are not aware how these aspects affect the health of your body and mind, please contact a physician of nutritional medicine or a nutritionist who has studied these modalities.

It's been a pleasure. Good health to you!

Always and with love!

REFERENCES

Balch, James F., M.D., & Balch, Phyllis A., C.N.C. PRESCRIPTION FOR NUTRITIONAL HEALING. (Avery Publishing Group, Inc.: New York), 1990.

Barnes, Carol. MELANIN (Protective Intoxicant Capabilities in the Black Human and Its Influence on Human Behavior), Vol. III. (Great Blackness Series: Texas), 1987.

Diagram Group (The). THE HUMAN BODY. (Facts on File: New York), 1977.

Hauschka, Rudolph. NUTRITION. (Rudolph Steiner Press: London), 1983.

Ornstein, Robert, & Sobel, Davis. THE HEALING BRAIN. (Simon & Schuster: New York), 1987.

Salaman, Maureen. NUTRITION: THE CANCER ANSWER. (Stanford Publishing Co.: New York), 1983.

Schmidt, Gerhard. THE DYNAMICS OF NUTRITION. (Biodynamic Nurturer: Rhode Island), (Rudolph Steiner Press: London), 1983.

Shelle, Orville. MODERN MEAT (Antibiotics, Hormones and Pharmaceutical Farms). (Vintage Books, New York), 1985.

GLOSSARY

AMINO ACIDS — The base acids and alkaline chemicals units of protein. The linking together of multiple amino acids creates a protein. There are (7) seven groups of amino acids from which proteins are constructed.

MELANOCYTE — Specific cells throughout the body that contain organelles which produce melanin.

MELANOSOME — Organelles located within melanocytes that produce and store melanin.

PHENYLALANINE — One of the eight (8) essential amino acids needed by the body to maintain healthy brain function and its an essential precursor to the production of melanin.

HALOGENS — A family of elements within the periodic Table of elements" that contain a unique electronic shell. Iodine and fluorine are elements belonging to this family.

L-CARNITINE — A substance found throughout the body and highly concentrated in the muscle cells to aid the cell in the oxidation (breakdown of fat).

L-CYSTEINE — An amino Acid, a sulphur containing amino Acid which can be produced by the body. It is prominent in hair, hoofs, and the keratin of the skin.

L-LYSINE — An essential amino Acid necessary for proper growth and development. Supports the body's resistance to viral infections.

L-METHIONINE — Essential amino acids required by the body to synthesize chlorine, the chemical base for the formation of the sex hormones and creatinine.

L-TYROSINE   A conditionally dispensable amino Acid that is a primary precursor to the production of melanin.

SUPEROXIDE DISMUTASE   A potent antioxidant that neutralizes the tonic effects of free radical formed by the body during its metabolic process.

BOTIN   A member of the "B" vitamin family synthesized by micro-organisms within the human gastrointestinal tract. It is important in the maintenance of the integrity of the hair and nails.

VITAMIN B_6 (PYRIDOXIN) A coenzyme needed by the body to metabolize protein and to synthesize unsaturated fatty acids. This vitamin is necessary for proper growth and development.

VITAMIN B_{12}   (Cyanocobalamine) A member of the "B" vitamin family, essential for the biosynthesis of nucleic acids and nucleoproteins for DNA and RNA synthesis. The body requires this vitamin for nerve tissue metabolism. it is primary stored in the liver and is a primarily melanin pigment.

PARA-AMINOBENZOIC ACID known as PABA, and is a form of folic acid needed by the body to neutralize free radical byproducts after tissue exposure to UV light and radiation. This vitamin is very important because it protects the skin from harmful light exposure.

MOLYBDENUM   An important element associated with many primary metabolic reactions of the body requiring copper and sulphur (sulfate) activity.

GERMANIUM Ge_{32} An important nutrient of vegetable origin found to activate and stabilize the immune system. It increases activation of neutrophils, "T" and "B" lymphocytes of the body.

CHLORINE A member of the "B' vitamin family and is a precursor of acetylcholine.

ACETYLCHOLINE A parasympathetic chemical mediator for nerve impulses.

COENZYME A nonprotein organic molecule required by an enzyme to catalyze a biological reaction. When the enzyme requires a CoEnzyme to activate a reaction, the combination of the Enzyme and CoEnzyme is known as a haloenzyme. Most enzymes contain primary melanin pigment vitamins to help activate the biological reaction.

BIOFLAVANOIDS A group of nutrients which are a byproduct of vitamin C, needed for the maintenance of arterial wall integrity. Important for tissue healing.

HESPERIDIN A co-factor of vitamin C found to be important in the maintenance and repair of arterial-venous tissue. It helps to regulate clotting factor of the blood.

RUTIN A co-factor of vitamin C found to be important in the process of wound healing.

FOLIC ACID A member "B" vitamin family essential for the synthesis of nucleic and the formation of healthy red blood cells..

THIAMINE (B1) A member of the "B" vitamin family which functions as a coenzyme in the major reaction that converts sugar into energy and water

RIBOFLAVIN (B2) A member of the "B" vitamin family, known as the "Anti Beriberi, Antineuretic" vitamin. This vitamin is needed for healthy nerves, heart, and digestion. This is a primary melanin pigment.

NIACIN	A member of the "B" vitamin family required by the body in the digesting of fats. Plays an important role in sinus, mucous membrane, and eye tissue health.
NIACINAMIDE	An "amino" of Niacin, important in fat synthesis, tissue respiration, and sugar metabolism.
PELLAGRA	A di-sease created by Niacin deficiency. The primary symptoms are severe skin rash, diarrhea, loss of memory, sore mouth, and inflamed tongue.

BIOGRAPHY

"In the creator of all universes we trust, perfect health is our birthright."

Dr. Jewel Pookrum

Dr. Pookrum graduated from Roosevelt University in Chicago. in 1968 where she completed graduate work in clinical microbiology and from Crighton University Medical School in Omaha, Nebraska in 1975, and completed her surgical internship in 1976. She then completed her Obstetrics-Gynecology residency at Henry Ford Hospital in Detroit, where she remained on staff from 1979-1981. She Received her Ph.D. in nutrition in 1992 from the American College of Wholistic Nutrition in Birmingham, Alabama..

Dr. Pookrum brings a sense of vitality and boundless energy to her work. She is the Medical Director and founder of the Civilized Medicine Institute (CMI). CMI specialized in medical treatment though nutritional medicine, which creates a healing environment where clinical medicine and wholistic practices are combined in a highly individualized approach. Her treatments have helped patients to heal visible signs of cancer, erase aging lines and learn to live happy, balanced and pain free lives.

Dr Pookrum's wholistic philosophy incorporates her surgical and gynecological training and a ten-year odyssey into wellness therapies and techniques. "The capacity for health lies within the human body. The body in a barometer for assessing one's ability to live in harmony with his or her environment." According to Dr Pookrum, "Nothing in our world has the power to make us weak, sad or diseased if we adopt the proper attitude, diet and commitment to wellness. Each of us can live in infinite perfection."

Dr. Pookrum is an acknowledged leader in the natural healing movement. She was selected by Nelson and Winnie Mandela to be their consulting physician during their historic visit to the United States in 1990. She has hosted wellness talk shows on WCHB and WQBH radio stations in Detroit. She has conducted lectures for major corporations. Secondary educations institutes, colleges, medical organizations and churches. She has received high praise for her dedication to sharing her vast knowledge of wholistic healing techniques. She has been sited as one of the Outstanding Young Women of America: named by the Detroit News as one of Detroit's leading physicians; and has been honored by the Coalition of 100 Black Women.

ALSO AVAILABLE IN THIS SERIES

(Other publications by the author in the Ethnoconscious Health Series)

Vol. I: UTERINE FIBROID CLINIC MANUAL,

Vol. II: UTERINE FIBROID HOME TREATMENT SYSTEM

Vol. III: VITAMINS & MINERALS FROM A TO Z

Vol. V: PROFESSIONAL GUIDE
 (for the Uterine Fibroid Home Treatment System)

Vol. VI: UTERINE FIBROID SUPPORT GROUP MANUAL

INDEX

American
    melanin-dominant 12
acidophilus 89
Acidophilus Buffans 89
Agent Orange 25
albinism 45
Aluminum 119
amino acids 20, 131
amphetamines 25
Amphojel 119
Anemia 117
animals 50
anthropologists 23
anti-viral substances 26
arteries 1, 25
arteriosclerosis 85
arthritis 13
Ascriptin 119
aspartame 89
asporotate 108
avidin 89
Biochemical 2
biochemical reactions 22
Bioflavonoids 97
biological combustion 49
blue light 39
bone density 11
bone marrow 88
Bufferin 119
calcium 12, 109
Cancer apple 81
candidiasis 113
catalyst 23
Cataract formation 53
Caucasian teenagers 10
Caucasians 10
Celtic background 23
central nervous system 28
cervical dysplasia 93
chelation. 108
chemical reactivity 23
chemotherapeutic agent 121
CHLORINE 133
Choline 91
chrysanthemums 14
COENZYME 133
coenzymes 107
Cogentin 91
collagen formation 115
color filter 53
concentration 23
cones. 44
contact lenses 50, 52
convulsive disorder 94
cookware 49
Copper 116
coronary 13
corpus calossum 45
cortisone 83
cyclamates 90
deficient 22
depigmentation 22
diabetes 13
Diabetics 62
diabinase 67
Differences and Skeletal Mass 11
Dilantin 94
DNA 43
Dog Star 45
Dogon tribe 45
Douche 119
Downs Syndrome 125

Index

ectoderm 27
electrical charge 23
electrical impulses 46
electromagnetic energy 21
electromagnetic spectrum 50
electrons 21
embryonic development 27
endocrine system 47
eriodictyon 97
Ester C. Polyascorbate 64
ethnicity 69
Eumelanin 23
eyeball 44
eyeglasses 50
Fair-skinned 51
fats 25
fatty acids 25
feedback mechanism 65
fibrocystic breast 72
filtered sunlight 51
fluorescent 37, 49, 53
flushing. 82
folic acid 93
food toxins 50
free radicals. 72
full spectrum 50
full spectrum light. 55
full-spectrum theory 53
gamma 44
gastro-intestinal ulcers 61
Gelusil 119
Gene Vitamin. 84
genetic information 13
glandular system 56
glasses 50
glutathione 53
glycogen 74
gout 13
HALOGENS 131
hematocrit 10
Hematological Differences 10
hemochromatosis 113
hemoglobin 10, 113
hesperetin 97
hesperidin 97
homocysteine 85
hormonal 50
humans 50
hydrocarbon 51
hypertension 13
hypertensive 71
hypothalamus 33, 45, 46, 47
immune system 26
incandescent 48
Indian 43
Infants 9
Inositol 95
insulator 26
intrinsic factor 86
Iodine 126
Iron 10
Kemetic 33
L-CARNITINE 131
laser therapy 93
light 28, 44
light spectrum 47
limbic system 45
Maalox 119
macrominerals 107
malabsorption 12
Malillumination 48
marijuana 25
Massengill 119
melanated photoreceptivity 45
melanin 10
melanin's optimal activity 20
melanin-dominant 11, 50
melanin-recessive 50
melanin-recessive metabolism 20
MELANOCYTE 131
melanocyte deficiency 79
melanocytes 22
melanosome 23, 131

Vitamins & Minerals: From A to Z

melatonin 25, 34, 37
metabolic function. 28
metabolism 21
metabolism. 50
microminerals 107
microscopic level 21
microvascular atherosclerosis 53
Minerals 107
mucus membranes 77
Mylanta 119
nanometers 48
nerve ganglion 34
nervous system 27, 47
neuroendocrine transducers 33
neurohormones 36
neuroleptics 25
neurologic dysfunction 37
neutralize radiation 27
NIACIN 134
nicotine 81
night blindness 61
nightshade 81
nocturnal melatonin secretions 38
NutraSweet 89
nutritional 10
nutritional assessment. 10
nutritional substances 25
obesity 13
optic nerve 34
Orotated minerals 108
orotic acids 108
osteodystrophies 12
osteoporosis 12, 74, 109
Oxalic acid 110
oxidation reduction reactions. 27
oxygenation 113
ozone layer 50
PABA 96
pantothenic acid 22

Para-aminobenzoic acid 96
paraquats 25
Parkinson's disease 91
pernicious anemia 86
peroxidation 72
phenothiazine toxicity 91
phenylalanine 22, 24, 131
pheo-melanin 23
photo receptors 44
photoreceptors 46
phytates 115
pigmented 50
pineal 33
pineal gland 45
pituitary glands 33, 45
planet 86
Plants 50
pregnant 10
premenstrual syndrome 72
prenatal vitamins 74
protein 12
protein-calorie 12
pseudo-melanin. 23
psychotic hallucinogens 25
psychotropic medication 91
Pyrex 49
Pyridoxine 84
pyrodoxine 22
quantum 48
quercetin 97
radiant heat 21
radiation 51
radio frequencies 49
rectal cancer 67
reproductive organs 36
Resonance 21
RIBOFLAVIN 133
rodopsin 45
rods 44
Rudolph Steiner 82
rutin 97
saccharin 89

Index

Sacred Triangle 33
saturated bonds 25
schizophrenia 37
seborrheic dermatitis 89
Selenium 118
serotonin 34
serotonin. 25
Serum melatonin 38
Sirius 45
skeletal 11
skeletal structures 13
*skeletalized 11
solanaceae 81
Sources for Protein and Minerals for Melanin-Dominant Individuals 12
steroids 83
sulfur drugs 67
Summer Eve 119
sun glasses 50
sunlight 48
sunlight lenses 52
Sweet and Low 89
synergistically 64
synthetic melanin 26
tardive dyskinesia. 91
teeth 13
tetracycline 25
Thiazide diuretics 70
third ventricle 33
Thomas Edison 48
thrombophlebitis, 97
tinted contact lenses 50
tinted lens 50
Toxicity 70
tranquilizers 25
tryptophan 25, 79
tyrosine 22, 25
ultraviolet 50
ultraviolet radiation 50
ultraviolet radiation. 27
Vanquish 119

vegetables 24
visible spectrum 44
visual cortex 46
Vitamin A 61
Vitamin B12 (cyanocobalamin) 86
Vitamin B5 83
VITAMIN B6 (PYRIDOXIN) 132
Vitamin C 64
VITAMIN C (Ascorbic ACID) 64
Vitamin D 69
Vitamin E 72
Vitamin K 74
vitiligo 117
Welsh groups 23
X-ray 11, 44
YAHWEH 5
zinc 67

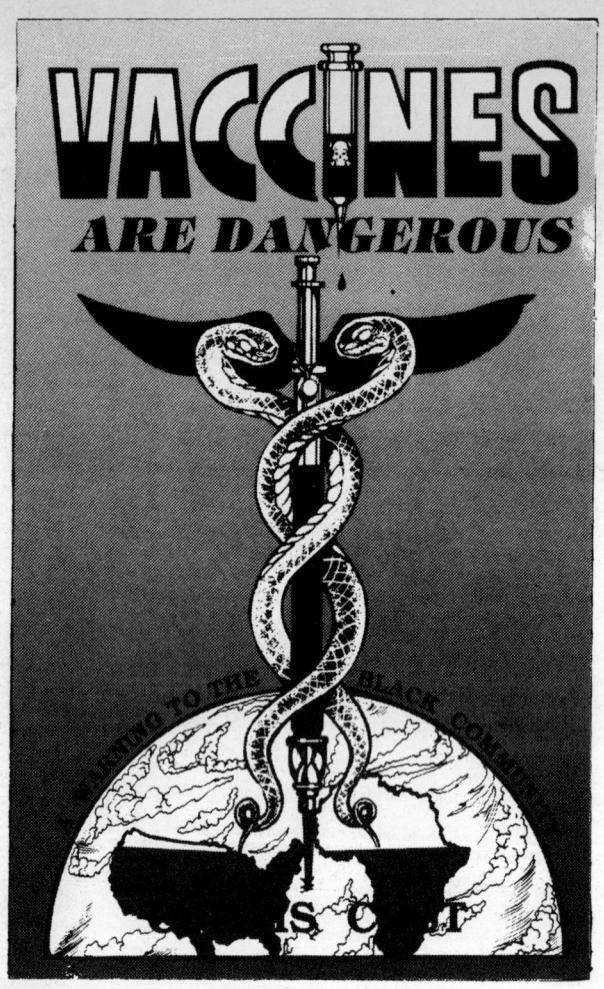

Vaccines Are Dangerous is a much needed treatise on an aspect of medicine that had been fraudulent from the onset. As a licensed physician within the United States and broad. I have observed the herd mentality of doctors, create the avenues and roads which have allowed the public to wander through. meeting their dis-ease and destruction.

Jewel Pookrum M.D.

To Place your Order See Back Page

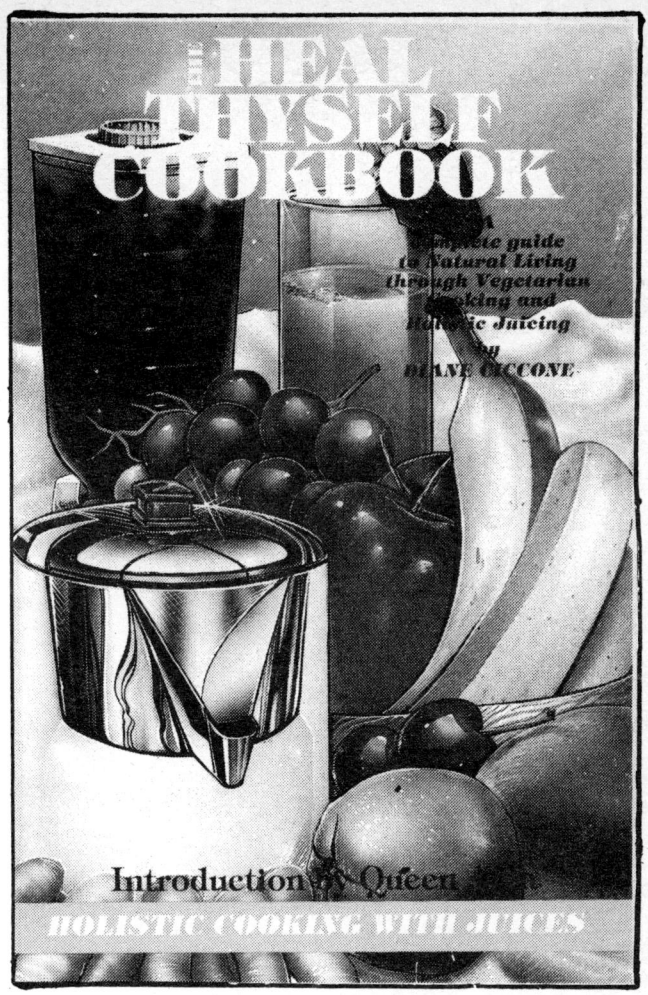

So much present day anger, stress and premature aging derives from our constant daily intake of fast foods, man-made processed foods and devitalized foods On the other hand by consuming natural foods of fresh fruit, vegetables, whole grains, seeds, nuts and live juices, along with specific herbs and spices, we are able to experience joy, peace, harmony , longevity, vitality and a body free of dis-ease. For you see, "We ar e truly what we eat"

Queen Afua

To Place your Order See Back Page

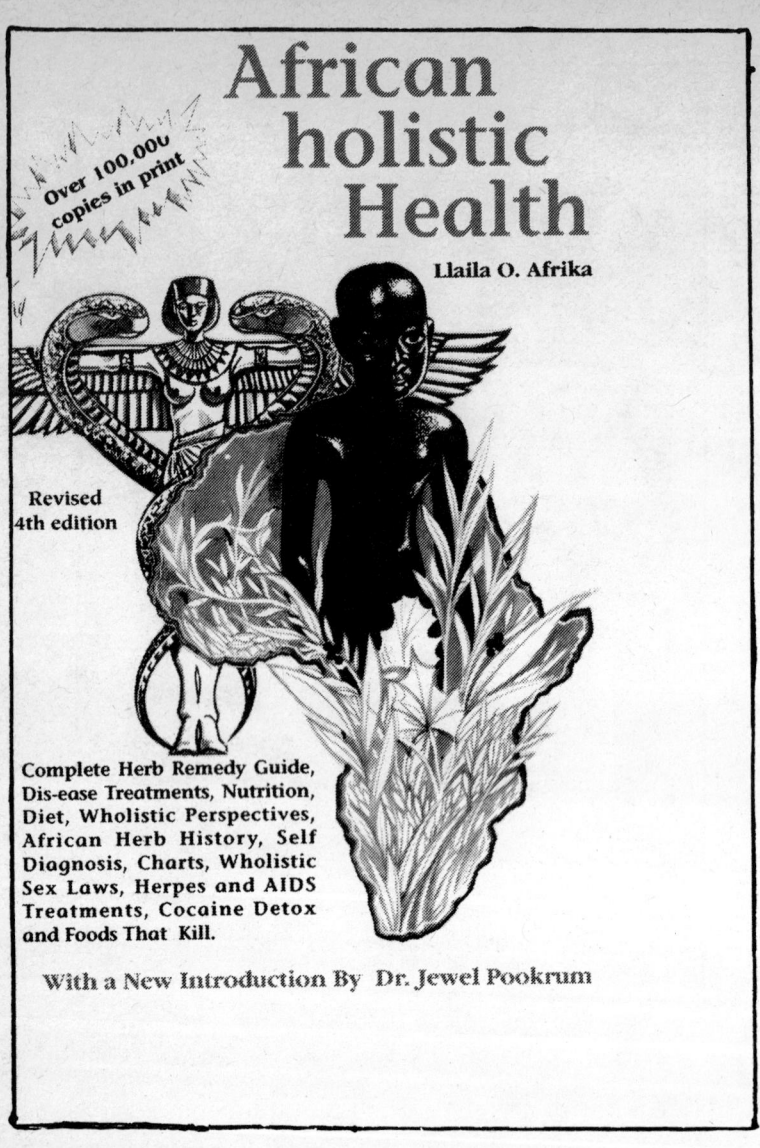

African holistic Health

Llaila O. Afrika

Over 100,000 copies in print

Revised 4th edition

Complete Herb Remedy Guide, Dis-ease Treatments, Nutrition, Diet, Wholistic Perspectives, African Herb History, Self Diagnosis, Charts, Wholistic Sex Laws, Herpes and AIDS Treatments, Cocaine Detox and Foods That Kill.

With a New Introduction By Dr. Jewel Pookrum

This book is the first of its kind on African Holistics. It provides a wealth of information that has been missing in Health, History, Social Science and Holistics. A masterpiece, a must for all learned people and a plus for those interested in learning more.

Dr. Bernard Matthews
Center for Natural Health
Detroit, Michigan.

To Place your Order See Back Page

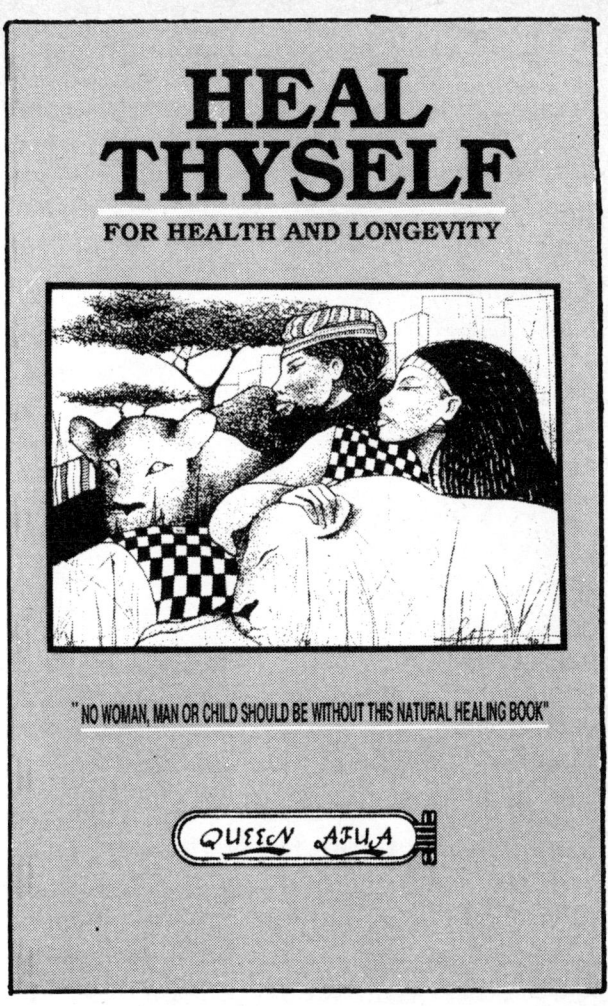

When you fast you find out very quickly why you wear "The Crown" To know thyself, heal thyself and be thyself in 21 days is an opportunity no one can pass up. Let Mind, Body and Soul come together and you will realize why life is the ultimate trip once you've learned to experience it.

Imhotep Gary Byrd.
Radio Personality W.L.I.B.

To Place your Order See Back Page

SELECTED TITLES *from A&B Books*

Title	Price
Blackmen say Goodbye to Misery	10.00
Education of the Negro	9.95
Heal Thyself	9.95
Heal Thyself Cookbook	9.95
Vaccines are Dangerous	9.95
Columbus and the African Holocaust	10.00
Columbus Conspiracy	11.95
Dawn Voyage	11.95
Aids the End of Civilization	9.95
Gospel of Barnabas	8.95
African Discovery of America	10.00
Gerald Massey's Lectures	9.95
Historical Jesus and the Mythical Christ	9.95
First Council of Nice	9.95
Arab Invasion of Egypt	14.95
Anacalypsis (set)	40.00
Anacalypsis Vol. 1	25.00
Anacalypsis Vol. 11	20.00
Document of West Indian History	14.95
History of the People of Trinidad & Tobago	14.95
The Negro in the Caribbean	11.95
Lost Books of the Bible	9.95

Mail to A&B BOOKS 149 LAWRENCE STREET NEW YORK 11201
TEL: (718) 596-3389 · FAX (718) 596-0968
$ 2.00 first book $ 1.00 each additional book. NY & NJ residents add sales tax.
Please find enclosed check/money order for $_____

Name:_____
Address:_____
City:_____ ST_____ Zip_____
Card Type:_____
Card Number:_____ Exp____/____

We accept *VISA MASTERCARD AMERICAN EXPRESS & DISCOVER*

NOTES

Perfect health is our birthright.

NOTES

Perfect health is our birthright.

NOTES

Perfect health is our birthright.

NOTES

Perfect health is our birthright.